MW01609871

WELLNESS
WAKE-UP CALL

by Dr. David Barczyk

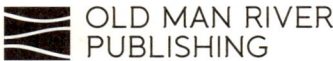 OLD MAN RIVER
PUBLISHING

Wellness Wake-Up Call
Copyright © 2013 by David Barczyk
All !N Wellness is a trademark of David Barczyk

Special discounts on bulk quantities of Old Man River Publishing™ books are available to corporations, professional associations and other organizations. For details, contact the Director of Book Sales at Old Man River Publishing™.

www.oldmanriverpublishing.com

Edited by Stacey Chamberlain, Camille LaHaye, Elizabeth Lyons, Jan Risher and Marsha Sills
Cover art, book design and illustrations by Lindsay Dreher
Photography of David Barczyk by Tim Landry
Printed in China

All rights reserved. No part of this publication may be reproduced, distributed or transmitted in any form or by any means, including photocopying, recording or other electronic or mechanical methods, without the prior written permission of the publisher, except in the case of brief quotations embodied in critical reviews and certain other noncommercial uses permitted by copyright law. For permission requests, write to the publisher, addressed, "Attention: Permissions Coordinator," at the address below.

Visit www.allinwellness.com for more information.

Requests for information should be addressed to:
Old Man River Publishing™, Lafayette, Louisiana 70508

Barczyk, David, 1969 -
Wellness Wake-up Call/David Barczyk – 1st edition
1. Wellness   2. Health

FIRST EDITION
April 2014

In memory of my dad. In life, he taught me to rely on myself and that working hard was best—not with words, but with action. In death, he taught me not to take today for granted.

— David

Advance praise for *Wellness Wake-up Call*

"Having dedicated my life to joining those who are crusading to bring answers that work to people looking to walk away from weight related problems and their associated unnecessary medical interventions, I have spent thousands of hours studying those research-based, cutting edge answers, and I have helped thousands of people use them to create lives of fitness, wellness, and optimal health. Dr. Barczyk delivers these cutting-edge answers in a way that could literally transform your life in ways that transcend just living life at a healthy weight. It is our thinking that drives our behavior, and Dr. Barczyk, through this book, can greatly help you to address this critical aspect of health while addressing comprehensively the aspects of our lives that can otherwise, unbeknownst to us, erode our health."

Robert Lecky, MD
Health Coach

CONTENTS

PROLOGUE

With few exceptions, the human body is a self-healing organism and would function without a hiccup if we were able to give it all the things it needs — nutrition, exercise, social and spiritual food. Most of the time, however, life gets in the way. The good news is that we all have the chance to make right with our physical, emotional and spiritual selves and live in a way that allows our bodies to function better. For those headed in the wrong direction — whether it's by living a sedentary lifestyle, with obesity or social isolation — change is within reach. We choose who we want to be every day. We choose how hard we want to work. We choose our reaction to adversity.

On the contrary, we also choose not to eat right, exercise enough or make destructive choices socially and spiritually. Inaction is a choice. To reverse a downward spiral and get life back on track, a person has to make a choice to live differently. The bottom line is that major lifestyle changes are almost always prompted by a Wellness Wake-up Call that comes in one form or another.

The idea of this book is that Wellness Wake-up Calls don't have to be organic moments inspired, perhaps, by an upcoming class reunion. Wellness Wake-up Calls can be intentional. The scenarios presented at the beginning of each chapter should act as simple barometers to reveal your level of wellness or alert you to a potential problem. How you do on the wake-up call is intended to guide and motivate you to make better choices about your health and lead to possible changes in your lifestyle. Each chapter is full of documented data, ideas for exercises, activities or simple lifestyle changes to support wellness.

Wellness Wake-up Call is based on years of research, both academic and practical. I believe most health issues can be traced back to some form of not living right. Of course, there are exceptions — and those unfortunate instances are not the ones addressed here. My personal devotion to wellness comes largely from the events of my childhood. My dad, an electrical engineer for AT&T, lived his young adulthood in the throes of the rat race of the Northeast corridor — commuting an hour-plus each way and focusing most of his energies on making a living. He was an introvert. A strong silent type, he never really communicated much. He must have internalized it all.

The stress of his life hit him with a stroke in his early '40s. Eventually, he recovered from the stroke. But by his mid-40s, he was diagnosed with a brain tumor, which was removed. He quasi-recovered from the tumor, only to have a degenerative neuropathy of his brain. His health steadily deteriorated for the next five years, until he passed away. He was and still is a major motivating factor in my life. He did what he felt he had to do to provide for his family.

Through his sickness, my mom was the primary caretaker. As aRegistered Nurse, she never hesitated in caring for him at home. She basically went from caring for her dad, my grandfather, who died of lung cancer, to caring for my father. We all helped — my sister, brother and myself. My older brother did what he could, which was amazing because he was limited in some respects, due to the fact that he wasn't able to walk without crutches as a result of the cerebral palsy that affected his lower extremities.

One night when I was 17, I was carrying my dad to the bath. I remember that I could almost hear my dad thinking, "My youngest son should not have to carry me to the bathtub." I vowed to devote my life toward wellness and continue to live with a keen sense of urgency to improve my life and the lives of those around me. Even though we choose to live with an eye always toward making the best choices, I also believe that struggle is an essential element in life. A lack of struggle leads to weakness — emotionally and physically. Therein lies the risk of creating lives and lifestyles for ourselves that in centuries past would only be lived by kings and queens.

Beyond doing my best to live right on my own, I have created All !N Wellness™, designed to provide businesses health and wellness information. The goal of our company is the same goal as this book — to offer individuals knowledge, motivation and empowerment to improve their lives — physically, mentally and emotionally. While wellness is an individual decision, organizations with wellness programs have shown real success in reducing absenteeism by 19 percent.

According to the Wellness Council of America, employees who participate in wellness programs take an incredible 70 percent fewer sick days than those opting out of wellness programs — and logically, healthier employees save the company, the government and the taxpayers' money.

According to Sales and Marketing Management, employees who exercise as little as once a week incur health costs one half to one third lower than those who do not. The American Journal of Health Promotion reported that the annual turnover rate for wellness program participants of the Canada Life Assurance Company of Toronto was 1.8 percent, compared to the companywide average of 18 percent. Incentive Magazine reported that Union Pacific Railroad found that 80 percent of its workers believed the company's exercise program helped to increase their productivity, and 75 percent believed that regular exercise was helping them to concentrate better at work.

According to the Association for Fitness in Business, NASA reported a 12.5 percent increase in productivity attributed to their fitness program. Participants were able to improve their work performance, as well as enhance their concentration and decision-making powers.

The timing of this book is crucial. With the federal government passing The Affordable Care Act, citizens have more reasons than ever to decide on their own to improve their health, but I believe free will leads to the most effective change. An incredible 75 percent of our country's health care costs are for treating preventable illnesses. Now, more than ever, your decisions about how you live your life affects not only you, but those around you. Whether you agree with the new law or not, the fact is that wellness is more important than ever.

As you read this book, you may find that it covers some things that most people have not considered wellness, but our bodies work as a total system, and this book is an attempt to address wellness from all angles. This is not a diet book. Nor is it an exercise book. *Wellness Wake-up Call* addresses concepts that cover the trifecta: brain, body and spirit.

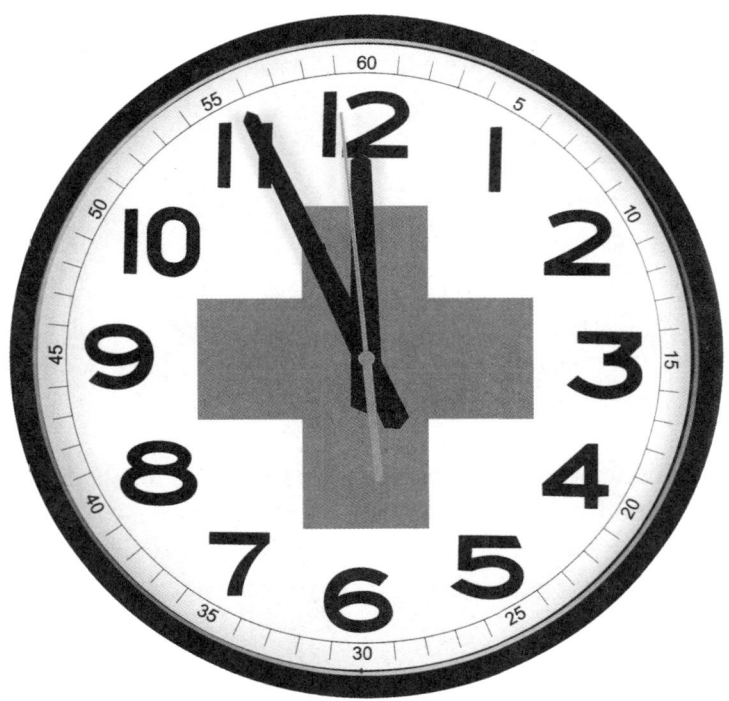

CHAPTER 1. Wellness Wake-up Calls

Wellness Wake-up Calls come in a variety of forms.

For some, it's the glimpse of a person they barely recognize in a photograph, prompting the question, "How can that be me?"

For others, the Wellness Wake-up Call may come during an attempt to perform some routine physical act that leads to a realization that what was once simple is much more complicated and may not even be possible anymore.

Whatever the catalyst, the fact is clear: A person who makes a major lifestyle change toward health is usually able to pinpoint the moment when he or she experienced a Wellness Wake-up Call.

The theory of this book is that Wellness Wake-up Calls don't have to occur organically. The following are simple tests, none requiring fancy equipment or special circumstances. Each can and should act as potential Wellness Wake-up Calls for readers.

Try them.

If you pass the first one with flying colors, move on to the next one. Try all of the Wellness Wake-up Calls to see if you're healthy all-the-way-around or which aspect of your life might need some work.

If you struggle with one of the Wellness Wake-up Calls, this book will show you ways to correct it. And that's the good part — it is correctable. If you're reading this book, you're taking a major step toward health. Now, take the next step, and try the first Wellness Wake-up Call. Based on your results, address your needs accordingly.

Try the suggestions in the book. They're simple and effective. Getting back in health doesn't have to cost a fortune or consume your life, but it is a choice you make every day.

Keep going with the rest of the Wellness Wake-up Calls. In fact, do them all, as each one addresses a different aspect of your health. Being healthy is about the whole body — body, mind and spirit.

You can be well again.

"You are the way you are because
that's the way you want to be.
If you really wanted to be any different,
you would be in the process of
changing right now."
— *Fred Smith*

If you begin and continue efforts toward better health, you have the potential to affect the health and wellbeing of others. In fact, if you have school-age children, your decision and subsequent actions will affect at least three generations for the good — yours, your children and your children's children.

You can pass on good habits — even the newly acquired — to your children who will subsequently teach them to their children. You're not just working out or eating right; you're changing the lives of future generations.

> "So many people spend
> their health gaining wealth,
> and then have to spend their wealth
> to regain their health."
> —*A.J. Materi*

1.2　Nature vs. nurture

Making healthy choices can do more than give you a better figure or physique. Making healthy choices may make the difference in you or the people you love acquiring a serious illness.

Surrendering to cancer, Parkinson's, diabetes or even ALS isn't a certain fate. In many cases, how you live — or nurture — plays a major role in whether or not illnesses develop.

1.3

In other words

If you need scientific proof, take a look at this: In a study released in 2008, North Carolina State University geneticists showed that environmental factors such as lifestyle and geography play a significant role "in whether certain genes are turned on or off." Basically, they were trying to determine the difference that nurture plays in the nature equation.

The scientists studied the gene expression of Moroccan Berbers, including nomads, mountain agrarians and coastal urban dwellers. Their conclusion: up to one-third of the genes expressed themselves differentially based on where and how the Moroccan Berbers lived. The scientists researched a specific group of people. This group of people (the Moroccan Berbers) shared similar genes. In fact, the scientists examined every gene in each of the three populations and found very few genetic differences. However, based on where and how each group lived, the genes developed different tendencies — leading to approximately 30 percent of the genes of the urban dwellers and mountain agrarians differentially expressed. The results led scientists to determine that environment plays a significant role in gene development, which means how you live affects how you grow and your health.

"Our growing softness,
our increasing lack of
physical fitness, is a
menace to our security."

—John F. Kennedy

1.4

Identical twins and epigenetic changes

Identical twins have long been used in genetic research to identify epigenetic changes — the changes that occur over a lifetime based on environment, like diet and tobacco smoke. Epigenetic changes are the culprits in the development not only of cancer, but also behavioral traits like confidence, shyness and fearfulness.

1.5

Not arguing the extremes

To be clear, there is no argument for extreme cases — sometimes people just get sick. Sometimes, both children and adults succumb to unpreventable and devastating diseases or genetic alterations at no fault of their own.

Human beings are all born pre-disposed to certain ailments. Which illnesses rear their ugly heads, however, is sometimes based on how each human lives his or her life. For example, if some people are born with a predisposed inclination to Parkinson's, ALS (Lou Gehrig's Disease) or multiple sclerosis, the expression of the gene doesn't have to occur.

For example, people who eventually get Parkinson's have the Parkinson's genes from birth. Something inhibits the expression of those genes throughout the person's life until the condition surfaces. As long as those brain cells continue to function, then Parkinson's will never express itself in that person. Through the course of life, traumas happen, accidents happen. Perhaps, the person makes poor decisions — albeit about diet, exercise or chemical exposure. Something they did or were exposed to allows the disease to show up.

ALS is the same way. In fact, most neurological and muscular disorders are the same way.

Living a healthy lifestyle decreases, but does not wholly prevent the probability of disease and illnesses. There are extremes. Sometimes a 9-year-old boy in a healthy environment and living a healthy lifestyle gets brain cancer, and no one can explain how or why such anomalies occur. This theory is not absolute and is about preventing what is preventable. Some things cannot be explained, but for those who'd like their best chances at long-term health, making healthy choices will decrease the probability of illnesses and disease.

"Genes load the gun,
but environment pulls the trigger."
—Dr. David Herber
(Director, UCLA Center
for Human Nutrition)

" To keep the body in good health is
a duty, otherwise we shall not be able to
keep our mind strong and clear."
—*Buddha*

CHAPTER 2.   The brain

Wellness Wake-up Call

Stand on one foot and see how long
you can balance. If it's less than 10
seconds or if you're wavering greatly,
that's a Wellness Wake-up Call.

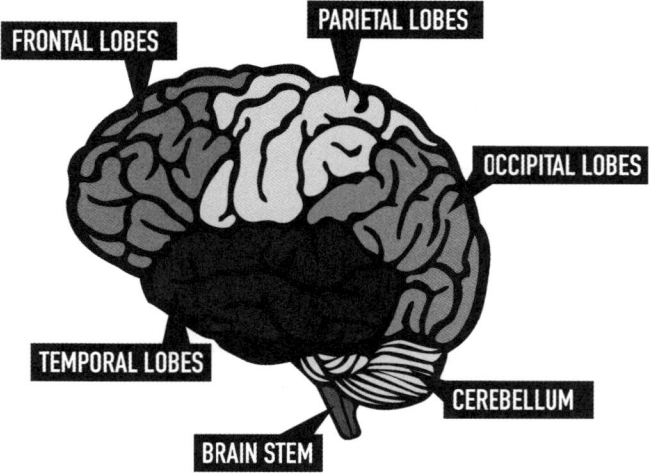

2.2

Use it or lose it

Have you ever given much thought to your cerebellum? Unless you're a neurosurgeon or experienced a brain injury (or love someone who has), chances are that you haven't.

Don't worry, you still don't have to understand how it works — or even think about it a lot. What you do need to understand, however, is that a lack of physical activity and movement causes the cerebellum to decline.

The bottom line is simple: if you don't get enough exercise, your brain stops working right.

"Lack of activity destroys the
good condition of every human being,
while movement and methodical physical
exercise save it and preserve it."
—Plato

2.3

The cerebellum

However, if you are interested: The cerebellum is a wondrous part of your body and brain worth knowing a little (or a lot) about. The cerebellum, called the little brain, has three primary functions:

- Maintaining posture and muscle tone
- Coordination of voluntary motor activity
- Maintenance of balance

With neural connections to other parts of the brain and peripheral parts of the body, the cerebellum continuously receives sensory information from all over the body — bones, joints and muscles — about their position, rate and direction of movement and the forces acting on them. It then tells the motor cortex what position a limb is in and what it is doing so the cortex can plan its next move.

The cerebellum also continuously receives information on the sequence of movements desired by the motor control areas of the cortex. With regard to movement coordination, the cerebellum behaves like a computer, constantly comparing the actual movement of the muscle groups with the motions intended by the motor cortex.

In case of a difference between the two, the cerebellum immediately sends signals to the muscle groups to correct the movement so that the desired effect can be achieved, much like computers calculating and correcting the flight path of airplanes or space vehicles.

Literally every voluntary movement of the body — and every movement's adjustment (up or down, left or right, faster or slower), although planned and executed by the motor cortex of the central nervous system, is regulated and controlled by the cerebellum.

"Let him that would move
the world first move himself."
—*Socrates*

2.4   The brain and its developmental timeline

Before birth, about 60 percent of human genes are dedicated to brain development.

In fact, a baby is born with 100 billion brain cells, called neurons. At birth, babies lose about half their neurons — a process sometimes referred to as pruning and may eliminate neurons that do not receive sufficient input from other neurons. The rest of the neurons are available and ready to make connections. Experiences during the early years profoundly affect brain structure and performance through adulthood. According to the Society for Neuroscience, connections diminish in number and are less subject to change after a period of time, and those that remain are stronger, more reliable and more precise.

Timing is everything regarding brain development. For example an injury (or deprivation) — whether sensory or social — that occurs at one stage of life may cause great damage compared to the same injury at a different period having significantly less effect.

The brain works in an interactive and integrated way. Specific structures are sensitive to language production and comprehension, as well as social/emotional responses.

In fact, research has demonstrated that if a monkey is raised from birth to 6 months with one eyelid closed, the animal permanently loses useful vision in that eye because of diminished use. This gives cellular meaning to the saying "use it or lose it." Loss of vision is caused by the actual loss of functional connections between that eye and neurons in the visual cortex.

Exercise, cognitive stimulation and being social can impact the number of cells in your brain put to good use and their efficiency by exercising diverse areas of the brain.

One of the most basic reminders of the connection between brain development and movement is a quick look at the major milestones of infant development — they are all linked to physical movement.

TIMELINE OF INFANT DEVELOPMENT

1 month — Lifts head while lying on tummy
2 months — Holds head up for short periods
3 months — Holds head steady
4 months — Can bear weight on legs and feet
5 months — Plays with hands and feet
6 months — Can roll over in both directions
7 months — Sits without support
8 months — Passes objects from hand to hand
9 months — Stands while holding on to something
10 months — Crawls well, with belly off the ground
11 months — Stands alone for a couple of seconds
12 months — Imitates wants with gestures

"All mankind is divided into three classes:
those that are immovable,
those that are movable,
and those that move."

—*Benjamin Franklin*

2.5   Did you know?

The reason crawling before walking is so important is that crawling usually represents the first action that simultaneously stimulates both sides of the brain for a child. That type of brain usage is called cross-extensor reflex. A baby has to move his or her left hand and right leg simultaneously — and then vice versa. Crawling is the action that begins the cementation of both sides of the brain working together.

Brain weight in grams

AGE	MALE	FEMALE
Newborn	380	360
1 year	970	940
2 years	1,120	1,040
3 years	1,270	1,090
10-12 years	1,440	1,260
19-21 years	1,450	1,310
56-60 years	1,370	1,250
81-85 years	1,310	1,170

(Data from Dekaban, A.S. and Sadowsky, D., Changes in brain weights during the span of human life: relation of brain weights to body heights and body weights, Ann. Neurology, 4:345-356, 1978)

"It is exercise alone that supports the
spirits, and keeps the mind in vigor."

—*Marcus Tullius Cicero*

2.6 Myelin — your body's secret to success

Myelin is an insulating layer that forms around nerves — including those in the brain and spinal cord. Myelin is made up of protein and fatty substances and provides a sheath around nerves that allows impulses to transmit quickly and efficiently along the nerve cells. The faster the impulses, the more efficient a human is at each aspect of life. Recent research has linked the breakdown of myelin to Alzheimer's disease.

According to a 2007 study published in *Alzheimer's and Dementia*, Dr. George Bartzokis, a UCLA professor of neurology, found that myelin loss promotes the build up of toxic amyloid-beta fibrils that eventually deposit in the brain. The fibrils become the plaque associated with Alzheimer's disease and will continue to destroy more and more myelin. The process disrupts brain signals and leads to cell death. "Myelination is the single most unique aspect in which the human brain differs from those of other species," Bartzokis said in the report.

Myelination in the brain grows strongly until middle age. The breakdown begins around the age of 50. Because modern medicine has expanded the average life span, as a species, this fact is especially important. Bartzokis compared how quickly a group of males, ranging in age from 23 to 80, could perform a motor task. He then correlated their performances to their brains' myelin integrity. Activity peaked at 39 years of age.

The research linked the speed of the task to the integrity of myelination over the range of ages. Because middle age brings decline in the repair of myelin in the brain, motor and cognitive functions begin to decline at an accelerating rate. Although the report seems less than promising for people over the age of 40, Bartzokis does offer hope. According to the researcher, preventive interventions, including physical and mental exercise and a healthy diet, could slow the process of the myelin breakdown. Bartzokis surmises that conscious lifestyle choices could even delay the onset of age-related disease, including Alzheimer's.

"Those who think they have not
time for bodily exercise
will sooner or later have
to find time for illness."

—Edward Stanley

2.7

Ways to lose brain cells

Brain cells shouldn't be taken for granted.

From cognitive learning to motor functions, the brain is the center of everything we do. Like a personal computer's RAM, brain cells determine how efficiently our thoughts and movements are processed.

A rogue computer virus can eat away at data and performance. Similarly, the wrong lifestyle choices affect our brain cells.

Everything we do — good or bad — has health implications.

To promote brain health, avoid the following:

Too much stress.
A little bit of stress is healthy. Stress keeps you motivated, and motivation leads you to achieve your goals. But when stress gets so severe that a person starts having adrenaline rushes, brain cells are at risk. The body is producing an excess amount of the chemical cortisol, and too much actually can kill brain cells. (Take a deep breath and try to relax after reading this.)

Sniffing inhalants.
Something as simple as the inhalation of paint fumes can lead to permanent brain cell damage. Some of the chemicals in inhalants leave the body quickly, but others stay longer and get absorbed by fatty tissues, including myelin, in the brain and central nervous system. According to the National Institute on Drug Abuse, long-term inhalant use breaks down myelin, which can lead to muscle spasms and tremors – or even permanent difficulty with walking, movement and talking. The effects can be similar to the symptoms of multiple sclerosis.

3 Recreational drug use.

Drugs are chemicals that tap into the brain's communication system and interfere with the way nerve cells send, receive and process information. According to the National Institute on Drug Abuse, marijuana and heroin activate neurons because their chemical structure mimics a natural transmitter. The drugs actually fool receptors and activate nerve cells, which incites neurons to send abnormal messages to the brain. Amphetamines cause nerve cells to release excessive amounts of natural neurotransmitters and can prevent the normal recycling of brain chemicals. The drugs lead to exaggerated messages in the brain – causing havoc with communication channels.

4 Concussions and other traumatic brain injuries.

A bump, blow or jolt to the head or a penetrating head injury can disrupt the normal function of the brain. According to the Center for Disease Control and Prevention, 1.7 million people sustain a traumatic brain injury each year. The severity may range from something as mild as a brief change in mental status or concussion to severe reactions, including extended periods of unconsciousness or amnesia, permanent damage to the brain or even death.

A Canadian study published in 2011 in the journal *Brain* found that athletes who suffer a concussion can experience a decline in their mental and physical processes more than 30 years later. The research looked at 40 healthy, former university-level athletes between the ages of 50 and 60. Nineteen had suffered a concussion more than 30 years before. Compared to those who had been concussion-free, the 19 participants showed declines in attention, memory and the slowing of some types of movement.

5 Eating junk food.

When your brain cells aren't provided with the healthy nutrients they need to survive, they starve and die. A study in the journal *Neurology* found that people with diets high in trans fat are more likely to experience the kind of brain shrinkage associated with Alzheimer's, and people with diets high in the B vitamins and vitamins C, E and D appear to have larger brains. Also, diets high in omega 3 fatty acids seem to benefit the small blood vessels in the brain and thinking abilities. According to the ongoing Oregon Brain Aging Study, people who had high levels of circulating trans fat had less brain volume and poorer memory, attention, language and processing speed skills. People with higher levels of omega 3 fatty acids were better with executive functions, including the ability to plan, problem solve, multi-task and perform other functions.

(6) Drinking too much alcohol.

Excessive drinking kills brain cells. According to the National Institute on Alcohol Abuse and Alcoholism, people who drink heavily over a long period of time may have brain deficits that extend into sobriety. The far-ranging effects can range from simple slips of memory to brain damage. Up to 80 percent of alcoholics are thiamine deficient, which can lead to the development of serious brain disorders, including persistent learning and memory problems and difficulty with walking and coordination. Long-term drinking damages the liver, which breaks down alcohol into harmless byproducts and clears it from the body. Prolonged liver dysfunction harms the brain, potentially leading to a fatal brain disorder that can cause changes in sleep patterns, mood and personality; anxiety and depression; shortened attention span; and problems with coordination. Some people even slip into a coma, which can be fatal.

(7) Dehydration.

Brains depend on proper hydration to operate. In a 2010 column in *Psychology Today*, Joshua Gowin states that dehydration can impair short-term memory function and the recall of long-term memory. Brain cells require a balance of water and various other elements to function. When people lose too much water, brain cells become inefficient. Without sufficient levels of water in the brain, ions get disrupted, which ultimately can lead to brain damage.

(8) Avoiding exercise.

The act of avoiding exercise doesn't kill brain cells, however, the effects that are associated with lack of exercise happen to be killers.

Exercise reduces stress levels, chance of brain damage and even creates new brain cells. If you are avoiding exercise, you happen to be setting your brain cells up for an early death. Exercise increases oxygenation to cells. It's never too late to get the oxygen flowing.

9 Smoking cigarettes.

In addition to being linked to cancer, lung and heart disease, smoking also may cause brain damage. A recent Scottish study looked at the effects of smoking on mental capacity over the course of 50 years. Dr. Lawrence Whalley discovered that smokers, all approximately 64 years old, performed worse on five tests that measured thinking abilities when compared to similar people who had either stopped smoking or had never smoked cigarettes. Whalley suggests that smoking might affect the oxidation process of the brain neurons. The brain requires a large amount of oxygen to keep the cells functioning, and smoking clogs the lungs and prevents oxygen from entering the system, which can cause premature death of brain cells and lower a person's ability to think. Smoking actually can cause a drop in IQ.

10 Exposure to pesticides.

In 2006, researchers at the University of North Dakota reported preliminary research indicating a link between pesticide exposure and neurological diseases, including Parkinson's and Alzheimer's. While most people think about exposure to pesticides through direct contact or indirect exposure through water or food, even the inhalation of tiny bits of pollen with traces of pesticides can carry dangerous levels of many chemicals. According to Dr. Patrick Carr, although the research is in its initial phases, there is clear evidence that pesticide exposure — even at relatively low doses — affects brain cells. The study finds that even small amounts of pesticides can damage or destroy the cells responsible for the reproduction of myelin.

11 Ingesting aspartame.

While some research finds no correlation between aspartame, the artificial sweetener found in many diet foods and beverages, and health risks, other studies are not as optimistic. A 2007 study done in Italy by the Ramazzini Foundation reports that rats fed aspartame had increased risks of various kinds of cancer. To avoid the risk, look for low-calorie, all-natural choices, like fruit, to satiate those sweet cravings.

(12) Lack of quality sleep.

We all know that when you don't get enough sleep, we cannot properly function the next day. Not only does lack of quality sleep interfere with learning and social functions (left-hemisphere), it can kill brain cells. To prevent brain-cell loss from lack of sleep, physicians recommend getting good, quality sleep every night. Some people run effectively on just six hours of sleep, while some need nine to keep a clear head. Find your own perfect level and be consistent.

(13) Having a stroke.

A stroke results from temporary loss of blood-flow to the brain. Usually, the damage from having a stroke is centralized in just one side of the brain. Strokes can cause anything from small lesions to widespread cell death. There are things people can do to reduce the risk of stroke. Lower stress levels, and stay active. If you do think you are experiencing the symptoms of a stroke, get help immediately. Millions of brain cells die each minute a stroke is left untreated.

"You will never find time for anything.
If you want time, you must make it."
— *Charles Buxton*

2.8

Ways to boost your brain

Want to improve your brain *(and your life)*? Try these:

Meditate.
Meditation, an attention-focusing process with Buddhist origins, has been known to increase IQ, relieve stress, and promote higher levels of brain functioning. Meditation also activates the prefrontal cortex of the brain, an area responsible for advanced thinking ability and performance.

> In 2011, findings in *Psychiatry Research: Neuroimaging* indicates that people who meditated for about 30 minutes a day for eight weeks had measurable changes in gray-matter density in parts of the brain associated with memory, sense of self, empathy and loss. MRI brain scans of the participants found increased gray matter in the hippocampus, the area associated with learning and memory. The scans also indicate a reduction of gray matter in the amygdale, the region linked to anxiety and stress.

② Creating art.
Drawing, creating pottery, painting and creating art in general stimulates the right-hemisphere of the brain and inspires creativity. Get out the colored pencils and begin drawing your way to a powerful brain.

③ Exercise.
Long-term exercise has been proven to increase brainpower and even create new neurons in the brain. Go out and get a natural high off of your own brain chemistry through exercise!

④ Avoid junk food.
Junk food has been proven to decrease energy in the body and promotes

brain fog. Cut some junk food from your diet, and reap the benefits of a more calm, focused brain chemistry.

(5) Deep breathing.

Deep breathing actually increases oxygen levels and blood flow to the brain. Ten to 15 minutes of daily deep breathing can improve the quality of your life and brain's functioning potential.

(6) Learn a new language.

Learning adds more structure to the brain and improves the brain's speech centers. Hablas español? It may be time for you to take a class or program to supplement your job skills and brainpower!

(7) Take fish oil or flaxseed oil.

Fish oil supplements are literally like membrane material for the brain. The two primary components of EPA and DHA each act to strengthen both the emotional center of the brain and boost focus. There is an increase in overall brain activity after taking fish oil for a while.

(8) Laugh it up.

Laughter causes a natural release of the brain's endorphins — chemicals that drown out pain and increase overall well-being. Laughter is a well-known, natural stress reducer. Watch a comedy, crack a joke and increase those endorphin levels!

(9) Engage in healthy debate.

Expand your communication network. Talk to lots of different people. Be willing to engage with people who may have different points of view. Don't attempt to persuade them to think differently, but be willing to listen to their different opinions. Just because it isn't your opinion doesn't mean it's wrong. Plus, a good, healthy debate strengthens the brain's ability to think quickly and apply intelligence to verbal situations. Work to build up your brainpower by engaging in plenty of healthy debate.

(10) Drink red wine.

Alcohol in moderation has been proven to be good for the brain. Why? It is rich in antioxidants — chemicals that actually protect the brain! One glass daily for women and two for men is generally considered a healthy amount.

(11) Eat healthily.

The food you eat might actually help brain cells regenerate. Researchers at the Salk Institute for Biological Studies in San Diego, California, are disputing the notion that the brain does not make new neurons as we get older. In a lab experiment, rats, equivalent in age to 63-year-old humans, were fed food high in antioxidants — including spinach, strawberries and blueberries. Surprisingly, the rodents actually showed signs of reversed age-related deficits in neuronal and cognitive functions. The rats' performance levels surpassed a group of similar rats that were not on the special diet. The participants showed remarkable stamina on neuromotor function tests, and they far outperformed their peers on tests of balance and coordination.

(12) Change your environment.

Do things on purpose that make you struggle. Don't look for the most comfortable route — even in something as simple as taking a different route home. To keep your brain properly stimulated, it is important to keep changing your environment. Drive a new route to work; eat at a new restaurant on Friday night. Changing the environment helps change the brain!

(13) Listen to music.

Learn a music style that's new to you — go back to the classics. It really does boost your brain. Studies have proven that listening to music strengthens the right-hemisphere of the brain and literally changes the structure. Those same studies have found that people who listen to music are generally smarter and have more emotional intelligence than those who don't.

(14) Better yet, make music.
Learn an instrument.

(15) Be empathetic. Be nice.
Remember how you feel when you help someone through a rough spot. Being empathetic and trying to understand the emotions of others is a skill that your brain can learn. Being empathetic is definitely a powerful trait to have and allows your brain to relate to the emotions of others.

(16) Think positive. If you are currently very good at thinking positively, chances are good that you already have a more powerful brain than those Negative Nellies. Take 10 minutes daily to think more positively and start noticing an improvement in thinking abilities and problem solving skills.

(17) Brainstorm.
A good brainstorming session to think of new, stimulating ideas is a great way to boost your brain's ability to think creatively. Brainstorming is actually a different way of thinking that will equip your brain with a quick creative boost.

(18) Write a letter or article.
Writing is linked to an improved memory and expression of thoughts. When you write, you are strengthening your brain's natural ability to convey thoughts and feelings. Writing is a great way to exercise your ability to analyze and build a thought process with critical thinking. Journals, diaries, blog entries and writing stories are phenomenal ways to fulfill your brain.

(19) Visualize.
Seeing yourself doing what you want to do is a very powerful thing. Visualize going to a movie theater. When the movie starts playing,

it's *you* doing what *you* want to do; being successful at whatever *you* want to do. Visualizing is another level of firing your brain in a different way. Visualization has been associated with focus at a deeper level. Many successful athletes that are able to play "in the zone" actually visualize their game at a deeper level. Visualization has been linked to lowered stress, increased creativity and peak mind-body performance.

20 Get some sleep.

If you're getting less than six hours of sleep, you're killing brain cells and at a higher risk of having a stroke. Sleep helps to clear out mental clutter and unimportant thoughts. Getting a good night's sleep can also be the difference between a sharp memory and feeling forgetful.

21 Do puzzles.

If you're a math person, do crossword puzzles. If you're a word person, do Sudoku.

22 Read books.

Reading books teaches your brain to adapt to absorb large amounts of information in shorter periods of time. Books challenge your thinking abilities and memorization skills, as well as boost vocabulary and critical thinking skills. Not only do you learn something from reading a book, but also your brainpower increases as you build up the book load.

23 Turn off the television — and electronics including phone, iPod, iPad or whatever else is the newest gadget du jour.

Watching television or sitting transfixed with an iPad may not be the way rotting begins in the brain, but such mindless activity is a key ingredient in the rotting process. A little television never hurt anyone, but it does definitely change brain functioning. The act of watching television slows brainwaves and causes a decline in brain fitness.

(24) Eat less.

Eating too much food has the effect of decreasing blood flow to the brain and increasing blood flow to the digestive system. Therefore, if you are able to cut back on the total amount of food you consume, you will have enhanced brain functioning. In several lab studies, rats on a calorie-restricted diet had increased blood flow to their brains.

(25) Eat breakfast.

When kids who hadn't eaten breakfast for a while began to eat breakfast, their math grades went up an entire letter grade (on average). Breakfast is probably the most important meal of the day — it provides your body with fuel for the rest of the day. If you don't have time to eat an entire breakfast in the morning, at least have some sort of snack. It could give your brain a powerful edge. *Refer to chapter on diet.

(26) Mimic others.

Being able to mimic other's actions and speech activates several areas of the brain that are usually inactive. Mimicking others, if done in a fun, playful manner, can improve your brainpower and the brain's natural ability to adapt quickly when faced with new situations. Mimicking can also give you a competitive advantage. An 11-year-old girl wanted to learn how to do a backhand, so she watched Roger Federer — and learned to do a beautiful single-hand backhand, as opposed to the typical two-handed backhand a teacher would have taught her.

(27) Have sex.

Not only is having sex a great way to naturally release vital hormones in the brain, it's also a great cardiovascular workout, and if you're having sex in a healthy relationship with one person, it's also emotionally good for you.

(28) Appreciate a variety of smells.

The olfactory evolved directly from the temporal lobe of the brain

— that's the area of human memory. Some smells, including basil, peppermint and lemon blossoms, are said to be good for your brain. Basil is used as a brain booster in aromatherapy and is one of certain fragrances that actually change brain functioning. Additionally, the scent of peppermint speeds up brain functioning.

29 Stay in school.
The more educated you are, the less likely you are to get Alzheimer's. Like it or not, being in school is good for your brain.

30 Ask questions.
Take a cue from kids with active brains. Asking questions helps keep your brain in shape.

"We are what we repeatedly do.
Excellence, therefore, is not
an act but a habit."
— *Aristotle*

> "Intellectual tasting of life will
> not supersede muscular activity."
> — *Ralph Waldo Emerson*

CHAPTER 3. Get up and move

Wellness Wake-up Call

When was the last time you sweated? I mean really sweated — not the face sheen that appears when you're in a hot environment or spend some time in a sauna. The question is: When was the last time you worked up a good sweat? If you haven't worked up and maintained 30 consecutive minutes of sweating within the last 48 hours, that's a Wellness Wake-up Call.

An Ideal Workout Regimen Includes:

- 10 minutes of warm-up
- 30 minutes of high activity/sweating
- 10 minutes of cool down.

3.2

Get moving

Americans are killing themselves — and playing a major role in bankrupting the country — by not getting up off the couch. Research shows that physical inactivity poses the greatest health risk to Americans. As many as 50 million Americans are living sedentary lives, putting them at increased risk of health problems and even early death, according to a leading expert in exercise science.

Steven Blair, a professor of exercise science and epidemiology at the University of South Carolina's Arnold School of Public Health, has called Americans' physical inactivity "the biggest public health problem of the 21st century." Approximately 25 to 35 percent of American adults are inactive, with sedentary jobs, no regular physical activity program and generally inactive around the house or yard.

"This amounts to 40 million to 50 million people exposed to the hazard of inactivity," Blair told the American Psychological Association. "Given that these individuals are doubling their risk of developing numerous health conditions compared with those who are even moderately active and fit, we're looking at a major public health problem."

The research comes from the Aerobics Center Longitudinal Study, which found that a person's fitness level was a significant predictor of mortality. In the ongoing study, which began in 1970 and includes more than 80,000 patients, the researchers periodically measured the participants' body composition and body mass index, and each patient underwent a stress test.

As the study progressed, researchers found that in the participants, poor fitness level accounted for about 16 percent of all deaths in both men and women. According to the research, the deaths could have been avoided if the people had only spent 30 minutes a day walking. The Aerobics Center Longitudinal Study also reported that moderately fit men lived six years longer than unfit men. Interestingly, women who were very fit were 55 percent less likely to die from breast cancer than women who were not in good shape. Blair also found a correlation between exercise and the mind, referring to recent emerging evidence that activity delays the mind's decline and is good for brain health overall.

According to Blair, doing something is better than doing nothing — and doing more is better than doing less. "We need numerous changes to promote more physical activity for all, including public policies, changes in the health-care system, promoting activity in educational settings and work sites, social, physical and environmental changes. We need more communities where people feel comfortable walking. I believe psychologists can help develop better lifestyle change interventions to help people be more active via the Internet and other technological methods," Blair said.

But sedentary behavior involves more than just a lack of exercise. Sedentary behavior pairs with a lack of whole-body movement as predictors of increased mortality and increased incidence of obesity, diabetes, heart disease and cancer, regardless of the level of physical exercise.

3.3   It takes more than exercise

Occasionally getting on a treadmill isn't enough. Sedentary behavior is more than just a lack of exercise.

According to an article published in the *British Journal of Sports Medicine*, Swedish researchers explain that sedentary behavior is chronic muscular inactivity. Elin Ekblom-Bak of the Karolinska University Hospital in Stockholm, Sweden, and colleagues argue that prolonged sitting is an independent risk factor for disease. According to the researchers, the body responds differently to prolonged sitting and physical exercise — and that long periods of sedentary behavior worsen the risk for disease.

Inactivity, which seems to be becoming a cultural trend in America, goes against thousands of years of human evolution. The human genome of today was sculpted and refined through generations based on human beings working daily for food. Survival required physical labor. People who worked the hardest and smartest flourished, further promoting the genes for the benefits of physical labor. Today's inactive and sedentary lifestyles run in the opposite direction of genetics. In a *Journal of Physiology* article, scientists claim "our current genome is maladapted, resulting in abnormal gene expression, which in turn frequently manifests itself as clinically over disease. We speculate that some of these genes still play a role in survival by causing premature death from chronic diseases produced by physical inactivity." The researchers speculate that genes evolved with the expectation of requiring a certain threshold of physical activity for normal physiologic gene expression.

In other words, daily physical activity is necessary to normalize gene expression toward patterns established to maintain survival.

> For most adults, the thought of exercising becomes about as much fun as ironing or having a root canal — but it doesn't have to be that way.

3.4   A slippery slope

According to the Surgeon General, more than 60 percent of American adults don't exercise regularly and 25 percent aren't active at all. Where do you fit in the mix? In 2012, two-thirds of American adults were considered overweight or obese (*Flegal et al, 2012*).

Think about your high school physical science class and think about Sir Isaac Newton. Remember inertia? Bodies in motion stay in motion. Bodies in rest stay in rest. Inertia is becoming the norm.

Remember when going outside to play was fun? When did physical activity become a chore? Psychologist Steven Bray of McMaster University decided to look at some of the factors that change people's relationship to exercise. Most children are more active than adults, and people generally stay active through high school. Bray found that college often was a stopping point for many people. The psychologist tracked 127 students and found that most freshmen participate in significantly less exercise that they did just a year before.

According to Bray, about a third of college students are active in high school and continue to stay active throughout the first year of college. Another third are active in high school and then let activity drop off. People who were inactive in high school tend to remain inactive. Bray relates the demise of activity to social changes. Many students who were athletes in high school aren't talented enough to play on college teams. They also become friends with people who already have adopted a more inactive life. People in other life transitions experience similar changes in behavior. Exercise often drops out of people's lives when they change jobs, move, get married or have kids.

"What it comes down to at each of these points is if we have the skills to be flexible and keep believing that these things are good for us ... I can keep it a priority and make it something I schedule the rest of my life around. Unfortunately, (exercise) is one of the first things that goes when we get busy with other things," Bray said.

3.5 Changing minds

If you don't enjoy exercise, you might be doing something wrong. Recent research has verified that there actually is such a thing as a runner's high. In a report in the journal *Cerebral Cortex*, researchers in Germany have found scientific proof that exercise can improve your emotions.

Using neuroscience, the research team documented a flood of endorphins to the brain during running. Endorphins bring mood changes — and the more endorphins, the better the runner feels. The study documents theories that have been out there for years. "This is the first time someone took this head on. It wasn't that the idea was not the right idea. It was that the evidence was not there," Huda Akil, a professor of neuroscience at the University of Michigan, told the *New York Times*.

Runner's high can now be measured. According to Dr. Henning Boeckner of the University of Bonn, who conducted the study, the discovery has interesting implications. The endorphins produced during running attach themselves to areas of the brain associated with emotions, especially the limbic and prefrontal areas. The same areas are activated when people are involved in romantic relationships. Boeckner is looking at whether the science could be applied to pain perception. "There are studies that showed enhanced pain tolerance in runners," he said. The research also could have implications for people who suffer from depression. Jim Blumenthal of Duke University has been researching whether exercise can reduce depressive symptoms.

Working with patients with major depressive disorder, Blumenthal divided his subjects into three groups — medication, exercise or a combination of both. After four months, the patients who had exercise alone showed as much improvement as the other two groups. Just more than 60 percent of the exercising patients no longer classified as clinically depressed at the end of the study, which compares to 69 percent of the patients who were only given medication and 65.5 percent of those assigned both.

Blementhal followed his subjects after the study and found that patients who exercised had half the risk of being depressed six months after the experiment as those who didn't.

> "Leave all the afternoon for exercise and recreation, which are as necessary as reading. I will rather say more necessary because health is worth more than learning."
> — *Thomas Jefferson*

3.6 Take a deep breath

Never take breathing for granted. In yoga, breath is known as prana, and it is considered a universal energy that can be used to find a balance between the body and mind, the conscious and the unconscious and the sympathetic and the parasympathetic nervous system. Did you know that breathing is the only bodily function we do both voluntarily and involuntarily?

When we are stressed, the sympathetic nervous system is stimulated. The heart rate rises, we sweat, muscles tense and breathing becomes rapid and shallow. Through voluntary breathing, you can change your body's reaction. By consciously focusing on your breaths, you can influence the sympathetic nervous system that regulates blood pressure, heart rate, circulation, digestion and other functions. Try to retrain your breathing. Chronic stress can restrict the connective and muscular tissue in the chest, which results in a decreased range of motion of the chest wall. With rapid and shallow breathing, the chest does not expand as much and much of the air exchange occurs at the top of the lung tissue near the head. This is considered chest breathing.

Place your right hand on your chest and your left hand on your abdomen. When you breathe, see which hand rises more. If your right hand rises more, you are a chest breather. Chest breathing is inefficient. Less oxygen transfers to the blood, which results in a poor delivery of nutrients to the tissues. But you can train your breathing, just like you can learn to play the guitar or drive a car.

By voluntarily making deep breathing a habit, you will find that you will begin to breathe from the abdomen even while you are sleeping. By breathing with your abdomen, blood pulls into the chest, which improves the venous return to the heart. The process leads to improved stamina. Abdominal breathing can help your body fight viruses and disease. It also improves athletic ability and gives you more energy. It even can put you in a better mood. Abdominal breathing stimulates the relaxation response that results in less tension and an overall sense of well being.

3.7   Don't get out of bed — just yet

We all have those mornings where just the thought of rolling out from under the warmth of a cozy comforter seems like a Herculean task. Instead of forcing yourself to get up and hit the treadmill, try a little compromise. There are a number of beneficial exercises you can do from the comfort of your own bed. The bed actually can be an effective place to perform both cardiovascular and strength exercises.

— Try this abdominal exercise. Lying flat, take a pillow and place it under your lower back. Put your hands at your side, palms down. Keep your feet together, and slowly lift your legs while keeping your ankles together. Tighten your stomach muscles and breathe in. Continue the inhalation while you slowly spread your legs apart. Count to five, and then bring your legs back together. Slowly bring your legs back down to the mattress. Repeat five times. Add more repetitions as you build up strength.

— Give the standard push-up a twist, and sculpt your arms and strengthen your core. Place your knees (or toes) on the bed and hands directly under shoulders, palms flat on the bed. Keep your back perfectly straight. Lower your chest to the bed, then return to the starting position. Perform as many repetitions as possible.

— Sit on your bed with legs extended in front of you and arms resting at your side. Bend your knees, and place your feet flat on the bed. Both your hands and your feet should be flat on the bed pointing in opposite directions of each other. Using a smooth action, press firmly into your hands and feet. Straighten your elbows and lift your hips up toward the ceiling to form a straight line with your hips. (Your body should look like a table.) Hold the position and tighten your butt muscles. Retract to the starting position. Repeat three times or add more as you get adjusted to the exercise.

— Lie flat on your back without a pillow. Stretch both arms to your side at shoulder length. Keep your arms and shoulders flat on the bed, and roll your head to the right. At the same time, lift your right knee to your chest. Breathe in while you tighten the stomach muscles. Breathe out as you roll your right knee and hip to the floor on your left side. (Don't press so far that it begins to hurt.) Breathe out as you slowly roll back to the original position. Roll your head to the left and perform the same exercise on the opposite side. Do the exercise five times on both sides.

"The only way for a rich man to be healthy
is by exercise and abstinence,
to live as if he were poor."
— *William Temple*

3.8   Add exercise to your daily life

Exercising 30 minutes a day is good for you. Exercising doesn't mean having to go to the gym. Be innovative. The creature comforts of our lives have led increasingly to sedentary lifestyle — more inventions have made too much of life too easy. Therefore, find ways to reverse the system and add exercise into your daily routine:

🕐 Park further from the store door and walk briskly.

🕐 Put up groceries at a non-leisurely pace — like it's urgent.

🕐 Take the stairs, not the elevator or escalator

Living life like it's urgent leads to a fuller life. Many people have the "I'll do it tomorrow" attitude that often leads to a less-than existence. Even doing mundane tasks like putting away groceries with urgency changes the pace of life and leads to more abundance.

You don't have to join a gym. Make daily tasks and chores exercise. For example, use soup cans to do lifts to the front and side. Use other household items, including towels for resistance in yoga or the garden hose for stretching exercises, to change your daily fitness level.

Find what you like. Don't do the same thing over and over again. Use YouTube, the Internet, a personal trainer, friends or ask your physician for new recommendations on different ways to exercise. Variety is the spice of life — even in fitness.

3.9   What is your heart rate?

An athlete has a resting heart rate of 45 beats per minute. The heart is a muscle. Like any other muscle, if it is exercised and efficient, it moves more blood by working less. If you don't ask it to work, then it doesn't really work. An average heart rate of a healthy resting heart for a non-athlete is 70 beats per minute. To calculate your resting heart rate, count your pulse for six seconds and multiply by 10 (or for 10 seconds and multiply by six).

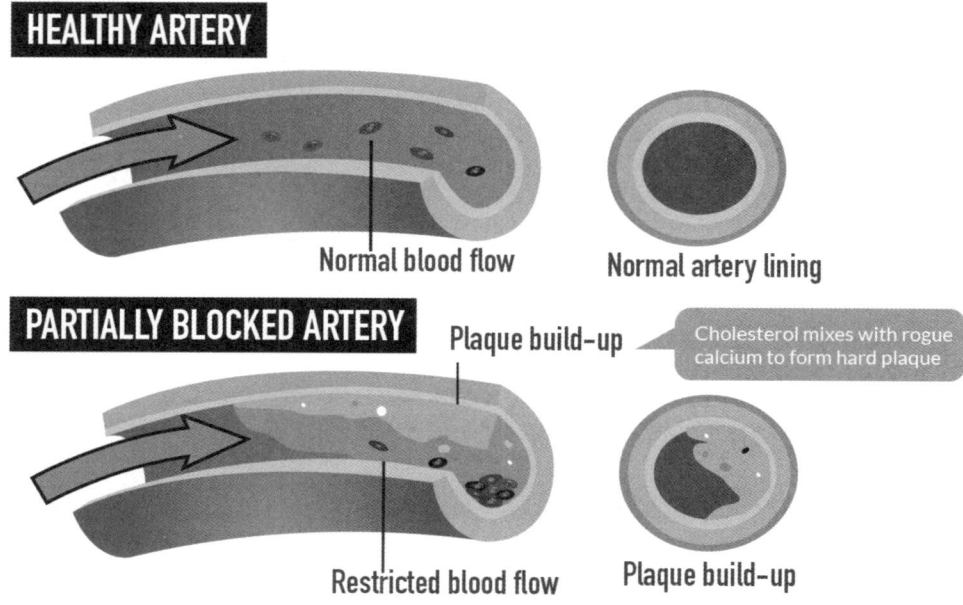

HEALTHY ARTERY

Normal blood flow

Normal artery lining

PARTIALLY BLOCKED ARTERY

Plaque build-up

Cholesterol mixes with rogue calcium to form hard plaque

Restricted blood flow

Plaque build-up

3.10 Understanding cholesterol's bad rap

On its own, cholesterol isn't bad. It's one of many ingredients our body requires to keep us healthy. Cholesterol comes from two sources: our body and the food we eat. In fact, about 75 percent of the cholesterol in your body comes from your own liver and other organs. About 25 percent comes from the foods you eat. In food, cholesterol is only found in animal products. Too much of one of the two types of cholesterol — good (HDL) and bad (LDL) — or not enough of the other can add to your risk of coronary heart disease, heart attack or stroke. A cholesterol screening measures the levels of both types of cholesterol. HDL helps keep the LDL from getting lodged in artery walls.

According to the American Heart Association, a healthy level of HDL may protect against heart attack and stroke. Low levels of HDL (less than 40 mg/dL for men and less than 50 mg/dL for women) have been shown to increase the risk of heart disease. Physical activity, including 150 minutes of moderate-intensity aerobic activity every week or 75 minutes of vigorous intensity activity usually helps your body produce more HDLs.

Many people inherit genes from their mother, father or even grandparents that cause them to produce too much LDL cholesterol. However, eating saturated fat, trans fats and dietary cholesterol also increases the amount of cholesterol.

"When it comes to eating right and exercising, there is no "I'll start tomorrow." Tomorrow is disease."
— *Terri Guillemets*

"Blessed are the flexible,
for they shall not be bent out of shape."
— Unknown

CHAPTER 4.   Get flexible

Wellness Wake-up Call

In a swimming pool or standing beside a chair, try to reach your right elbow to your left knee (by picking up your left knee and stretching your elbow toward it).

If you can't touch your right elbow to your left knee, that's a Wellness Wake-up Call. Either your body, muscles and joints have become rigid and inflexible, or your extra pounds make it "physically" impossible for the two to meet.

It's time for a change.

4.2

Wrong directions

In America, more and more middle-aged people have physical disabilities that limit their mobility.

According to the National Health Interview Survey, more than 40 percent of respondents ages 50 to 64 reported difficulty with at least one of nine physical functions. In a 10-year period, the study found a significant increase in the number of middle-age Americans who said that a health problem made it difficult for them to stand for two hours, stoop, walk a quarter mile or climb 10 steps without resting. Many also said they needed assistance with daily activities like getting out of bed and getting around inside their homes. The respondents often related the lack of mobility to health issues that began in their 30s or 40s.

A 2008 study in the health journal *The Lancet* estimates that as many as 5.3 million deaths around the world were caused by physical inactivity in one year alone. Not moving may be as hazardous to your health as smoking.

4.3

Natural changes

As humans age, the body naturally declines. Muscle mass, bone density, endurance, flexibility and balance all decrease.

According to the American College of Sports Medicine, beginning in the fourth decade of life, adults start to lose 3 to 5 percent of muscle mass every 10 years — and the decline increases after the age of 50.

Osteoporosis, a disease of low bone density that is largely preventable, affects 44 million men and women ages 50 and older in the United States — or 55 percent of that age bracket. The disease is responsible for more than 1.5 million fractures annually.

Although physical decreases are part of the natural aging process, they aren't unavoidable. Exercise can be a veritable Fountain of Youth.

4.4

Height-to-weight ratio

What's the best way to determine a healthy weight? You can look at your height and weight in the chart below to determine your ideal weight. Use the BMI graph on the following page if your current weight falls outside of your ideal weight.

Height	(Male) Ideal Weight	Height	(Female) Ideal Weight
4'6"	63 - 77 lbs.	4'6"	63 - 77 lbs.
4'7"	68 - 84 lbs.	4'7"	68 - 84 lbs.
4'8"	74 - 90 lbs.	4'8"	72 - 88 lbs.
4'9"	79 - 97 lbs.	4'9"	77 - 94 lbs.
4'10"	85 - 103 lbs.	4'10"	81 - 99 lbs.
4'11"	90 - 110 lbs.	4'11"	86 - 105 lbs.
5'0"	95 - 117 lbs	5'0"	90 - 110 lbs
5'1"	101 - 123 lbs.	5'1"	95 - 116 lbs.
5'2"	106 - 130 lbs.	5'2"	99 - 121 lbs.
5'3"	112 - 136 lbs.	5'3"	104 - 127 lbs.
5'4"	117 - 143 lbs.	5'4"	108 - 132 lbs.
5'5"	122 - 150 lbs.	5'5"	113 - 138 lbs.
5'6"	128 - 156 lbs.	5'6"	117 - 143 lbs.
5'7"	133 -163 lbs.	5'7"	122 - 149 lbs.
5'8"	139- 169 lbs.	5'8"	126 - 154 lbs.
5'9"	144 - 176 lbs.	5'9"	131 - 160 lbs.
5'10"	149 - 183 lbs.	5'10"	135 - 165 lbs.
5'11"	155 - 189 lbs.	5'11"	140 - 171 lbs.
6'0	160 - 196 lbs.	6'0	144 - 176 lbs.
6'1"	166 - 202 lbs.	6'1"	149 - 182 lbs.
6'2"	171 - 209 lbs.	6'2"	153 - 187 lbs.
6'3"	176 - 216 lbs.	6'3"	158 - 193 lbs.
6'4"	182 - 222 lbs	6'4"	162 - 198 lbs
6'5"	187 - 229 lbs	6'5"	167 - 204 lbs
6'6"	193 - 235 lbs	6'6"	171 - 209 lbs
6'7"	198 - 242 lbs.	6'7"	176 - 215 lbs.
6'8"	203 - 249 lbs.	6'8"	180 - 220 lbs.
6'9"	209 - 255 lbs.	6'9"	185 - 226 lbs.
6'10"	214 - 262 lbs.	6'10"	189 - 231 lbs.
6'11"	220 - 268 lbs.	6'11"	194 - 237 lbs.
7'0"	225 - 275 lbs.	7'0"	198 - 242 lbs.

Did you know that your waist size should be about half your height?

So, if you're 5' 5" tall, you're 65 inches tall, which means your waist should be about 32-33 inches around.

4.5 Body Mass Index (BMI)

You can find your body mass index (BMI) using the graph below. The body mass index is a measure for human body shape based on an individual's mass and height.

BMI was devised between 1830 and 1850 by the Belgian intellectual, Adolphe Quetele. It is defined as the individual's body mass divided by the square of their height. A healthy BMI rate should fall between the range of 18.5-25.

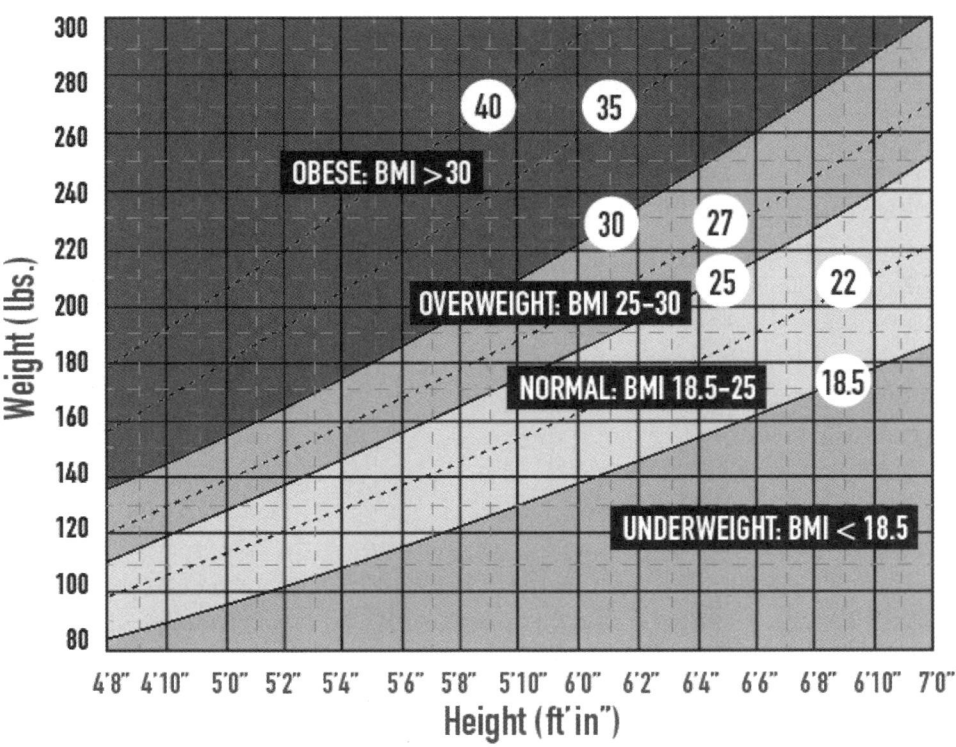

4.6

Turning back time

Even octogenarians can increase muscle mass.

Researchers in Boston worked with 100 male and female residents of a nursing home to see if weight lifting could improve their physical abilities. The participants, ages 72 to 98, lifted weights with their legs three times a week for 10 weeks. At the end of the study, the seniors showed impressive results.

On average, there was an increase in thigh mass of 2.7 percent. Walking speed rose 12 percent — and leg strength jumped 113 percent.

In a similar study of adults ages 65 to 79, people who lifted weights three times a week for three months increased their walking endurance from 25 to 34 minutes — or 38 percent.

And getting results doesn't require bulking up. Strength is as much about neurological patterning as it is about mass. The brain sends electrical signals via the nervous system to make muscles contract. This patterning can improve within days of starting a weight-lifting program. Neurological patterning was responsible for the 113 percent increase in leg strength in the Boston study.

> Pain syndromes are made worse by over activity and equally worse by under activity. For example, when it hurts to walk, many Americans choose to ride instead — or at the least park closer to the door at the mall, sometimes even getting a handicapped sticker...which leads to less activity, which leads to more weight gain, which leads to more pressure on the joints... big ball rolling downhill

Engaging in exercise programs also can help maintain endurance, which correlates to projected lifespan. In a study of more than 3,000 people between the ages of 70 and 79, statistics showed that the people with the slowest walking times had a higher risk of death. Another study found that men who walked less than one mile per day had a mortality rate that was more than double that of men who walked more than two miles per day.

Researchers who collected data on more than 41,000 men and women for more than a decade were able to analyze the relationship between walking and mortality. Men and women who walked 30 minutes or more per day had fewer deaths than those who walked less than 30 minutes.

Similarly, stretching and exercise are important to maintaining and improving flexibility. Some studies have found significant improvements through exercise in the range of motion of the neck, shoulders, elbows, wrists, knees and ankles.

Muscle training and exercise also can help improve balance. Decreases in balance as people age often leads to falls. The U.S. Center for Disease Control reports that one of every three Americans over the age of 65 falls each year. Among people between the ages of 65 and 84, falls account for 87 percent of all fractures. They also are the second leading cause of spinal cord and brain injury.

Exercise even has been linked to an increase in bone density. Researchers have found that weightlifting — and even walking — can increase bone density in the hips and spine. Physicians theorize that weightlifting causes stress on bones as muscles contract, which causes the bones to thicken. The impact of walking also stresses the bones and stimulates them to grow.

4.7   And the tailbone's connected to the...

On a macroscopic level, skeletal muscles are like levers. When muscles aren't used much, they contract and shorten. When muscles shorten, the lever stops working properly. Your body consists of multiple lever-type muscles. Even if only one begins to malfunction, it may affect multiple areas of your body.

For example, if the hamstring lever begins to shorten and malfunction, it affects the flexibility and function of your knee, which can affect the function of your pelvis, which can affect the function of your lumbar spine.

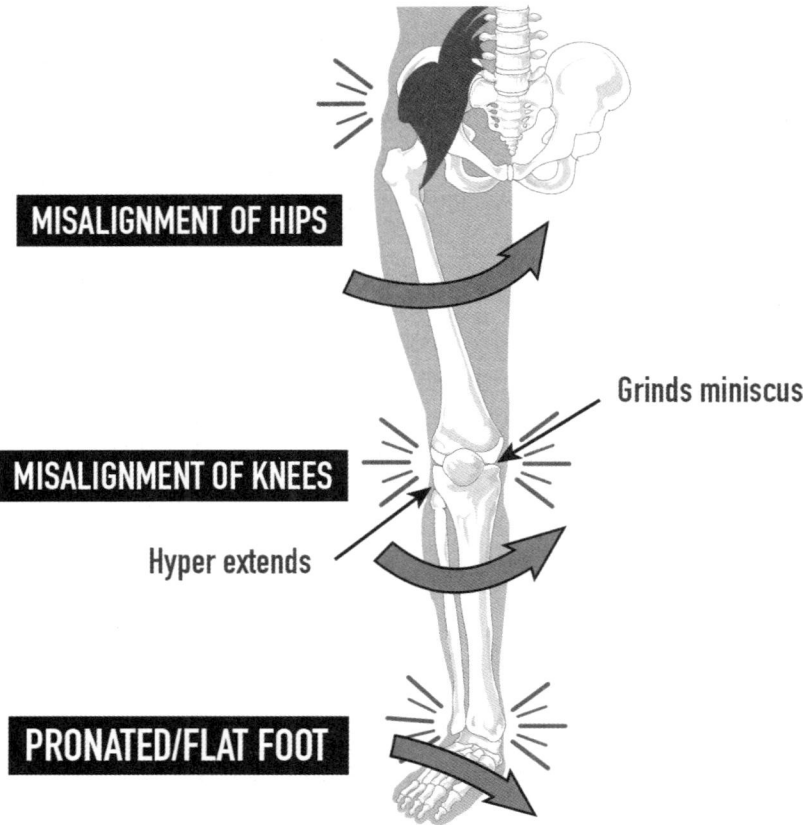

MISALIGNMENT OF HIPS

Grinds miniscus

MISALIGNMENT OF KNEES

Hyper extends

PRONATED/FLAT FOOT

4.8

Watch your posture

Most Americans spend the majority of their time in flexion, from the Latin word flectere, to bend. Flexion is a position made possible by decreasing a joint's angle. It is the opposite of extension. For example, the elbow is flexed when the hand is brought closer to the shoulder.

Most of the time, our necks are flexed. Our wrists are flexed. Our hips are flexed. We spend most of our time in flexion, as opposed to walking around, extended and opened up — which plays a role in general poor posture.

Posture is about more than pleasing your parents. Poor posture can strain the spine and cause backaches. Poor posture may compress the chest, ribs or lungs to cause breathlessness and a variety of other problems. Poor posture may compress the air in the chest and slow the flow of blood.

Poor posture is a problem.

4.9   Year-to-year, gradual weight gain — and it's consequences

Many adults who stop actively pursuing a healthy lifestyle gain about five pounds a year. Gaining five pounds in a year doesn't sound horrible, does it? However, think about the cumulative weightgain over a span of 10 years. That's 50 pounds. Over 20 years, it's 100 pounds. Significant weight gain is a silent predator that inches up on its victims.

Think about the gradual average weight gain in terms of a class reunion. A lean 120-pound high school graduate would weigh 170 pounds by the 10-year reunion. He or she would be a solid 220 pounds by the 20th high school reunion. Do you want to be that guy?

*"Let food be thy medicine
and medicine be thy food."*
— Hippocrates

CHAPTER 5.　　　Food and health

Wellness Wake-up Call

Check your pantry. If you have more than 10 items with labels on them, that's a Wellness Wake-up Call. If any of those 10 items has more than five ingredients in it, that's another Wellness Wake-up Call. If any of the ingredients are words you struggle to pronounce, there's your third wake-up call. And if you scored a Wellness Wake-up Call in all three — you've got a problem.

5.2

The future is now

Put down the doughnut. Drop the bag of potato chips — and dump the soda down the drain.

Everything you put in your mouth is linked to your future. The average American consumes close to 2,000 pounds of food per year. Breaking it down, that amounts to around 29 pounds of French fries, 23 pounds of pizza, 53 gallons of soda and 24 pounds of ice cream. If a person lives to be 80, they will have consumed nearly 68 tons of food during his or her lifetime — that's roughly 67,000,000 calories.

Whether you are 50 pounds overweight or a size 0, the food you eat is a crucial part of the overall health equation. Diet — defined as the foods we choose to eat — and exercise go hand in hand.

Without proper nutrition, your body can't function. Even the brain is affected by what you put in your mouth. Your brain is the one part of your body that actually can shrink from eating junk food.

The costs continue to creep due to the ever-widening American bottom.

As the seat sizes on Broadway, in planes, in stadiums and any other venue increase to accommodate for growing derrieres, seating density decreases — and who pays for that? The consumer, of course — no matter how large or small your derriere may be.

On Broadway, according to Theater Projects Consultants, the same floor space that could hold 20 seats in the late 19th century can only hold 10 seats today.

At the movies, popcorn isn't the only thing that comes super-sized. From 1900 to 1990, the width of seats increased from 19 to 21 inches. Since 1990, the seats have increased about 25 percent more.

A study in the journal *Neurology* found that people with diets high in trans fat are more likely to experience the kind of brain shrinkage associated with Alzheimer's disease. Conversely, people who have diets high in vitamins C and E, the B vitamins and vitamin D have larger brains.

People who have high levels of circulating trans fat have less brain volume, thus leading to poorer memory, attention, language and processing speed skills — and poor diet ultimately costs you money. Chronic disease that can often be reversed or prevented altogether by a healthy lifestyle, including proper diet and exercise, make up about 75 percent of the $2.8 trillion in annual health care costs in the United States.

5.3   Lose the fad diet mentality

Almost half of all Americans are on a diet, yet two-thirds are overweight and one-fourth have crossed the line into obesity.

A person is obese when his or her weight is 20 percent or more above normal and is considered morbidly obese when he or she is 50 percent or more above normal.

A large government survey, which actually weighed and measured people, found that about 5 percent of American adults are morbidly obese.
Dieting doesn't work. About 85 percent of people who go on diets fail. Although they may lose weight — even considerable weight, they rarely keep it off.

Maintaining a healthy weight isn't about following fads. You have to focus on what you eat. Changing your lifestyle and your relationship to food is essential.

5.4   Your drug of choice

A study in the journal *Nature Neuroscience* argues that high-fat, high-calorie foods — like bacon, cheesecake and ice cream — affect the brain similarly to cocaine and heroin. Compulsive eating habits resemble drug addiction.

But is food addiction real?

Science has begun to accept that sugar, fat and salt have drug-like qualities in how they activate the reward and pleasure centers of the brain. Like drug addicts, food addicts can develop a tolerance to food. No matter how much they eat, they are never truly satisfied. The craving is endless. Interestingly, infants are born with the ability to taste sweets, but the taste of salt is acquired.

When a food addict stops eating trigger foods (whether it's sugar or caffeine), he or she actually experiences withdrawal symptoms — including anxiety, agitation and physical reactions.

Do you:

- Eat more than you planned when you start eating certain foods?
- Keep eating a certain food even if you no longer feel hungry?
- Eat some foods to the point that you feel physically ill?
- Worry about not being able to eat certain foods?
- Go out of your way to obtain certain foods or drinks even when there are more convenient alternatives?
- Let eating get in the way of work, spending time with family and doing recreational activities?
- Avoid professional or social situations where certain foods will be available because of a fear of overeating?
- Have problems functioning at work because of food and eating?

"More die in the United States of too much food than of too little."
— *John Kenneth Galbraith*

5.5

Hooked on a feeling

Even people who aren't food addicts may have unhealthy relationships with certain foods.

Do you eat because you are hungry, or is something else inspiring you to open the refrigerator? Americans refer to some of the unhealthiest food available — from cakes and pies to macaroni and cheese — as "comfort food," and their consumption has more to do with emotions than nutrition.

Some people eat comfort foods when they are depressed, but comfort eating happens just as often to maintain an already good mood.

According to the Food and Brand Lab at the University of Illinois, ice cream is the top comfort food in America for both men and women. For women, chocolate and cookies follow close behind. Men's second choice is usually pizza, steak or casserole.

An *American Demographics* report found that specific foods are often linked to specific moods. When people are happy, 32 percent of the time they will emotionally eat with foods like steak or pizza. Sad people reach for ice cream and cookies 39 percent of the time, and 36 percent of people who are bored favor potato chips.

Emotional eating is about feeding a feeling rather than real hunger. For an emotional eater, the desire for food is triggered by something psychological rather than physical. Evolution is partially responsible.

Since the beginning of time, evolution has made everything about eating as rewarding as possible. At least one 2011 study examines the connection between volunteers' stomachs and brains, suggesting that hormones in our stomachs appear to communicate directly with our brains — independent of any feelings we have about a particular food.

In the study, performed at the University of Leuven in Belgium, volunteers were fed through unmarked feeding tubes. In a series of tests performed after participants were fed, those who received saturated fat appeared to fend off negative emotions more easily than those who didn't receive saturated fat.

Lukas Van Oudenhove, M.D., one of the researchers, suggests that the deep-seated connection between our stomachs and brains — which helped keep humans alive throughout most of history — may have outlived its usefulness.

"These days it may not be a good thing anymore," Van Oudenhove said. "When food is available anywhere, then it may be a bad thing, leading to obesity or eating disorders in some people."

While there's nothing wrong with the occasional comfort food, the problem lies when people lose self-control and self-discipline — and don't resist the temptation to feed an emotional need or discomfort with food. Physical hunger comes on gradually, but emotional hunger is sudden. It's all about filling a void rather than an empty stomach. Emotional eaters crave a specific food, like pizza or ice cream — and only that food will satisfy the need.

While someone feeling physical hunger can wait to eat, emotional hunger demands immediate satisfaction, and it is difficult to stop eating even if your stomach is full. Although emotional eating is about fulfilling a feeling, the eater often feels guilt at the end, rather than being truly satisfied.

Sound familiar?

> "I hid myself in food."
> — *Gordon Ramsay*

5.6 Back to basics

Why are most people's diets lacking in basic nutrition?

It's not for a lack of availability.

Although food from all the major food groups has become readily available since 1970, Americans still fall short of federal dietary recommendations. In fact, three-fourths of the U.S. population does not meet daily recommended dietary allowances.

The majority of Americans consume 22 percent of their total daily calories from what they drink, especially beverages sweetened with sugar or high-fructose corn syrup. Americans are consuming too many foods and beverages that are high in fats and carbohydrates and too few nutrient-dense foods and beverages, fruits and vegetables. According to a U.S. Department of Agriculture study, the average American over-consumes refined grains yet falls short on whole-grain intake.

Although dietary guidelines recommend people eat 2 cups of fruit and 2 ½ cups of vegetables per day, the average person eats less than a cup of fruit and only about a cup and a half of vegetables. Americans also are over-consuming in the meat, eggs and nuts category. Instead of taking in 5.5 ounces per day, the average person eats 6.5 ounces, often favoring red meat.

Sugars and sweeteners may be the worst offenders.

Although guidelines warn of the danger of consuming more than 8 teaspoons a day, Americans consume an average of 30 teaspoons a day — and many Americans ingest even more.

So what should you be eating?

The perfect diet is low in unhealthy carbohydrates (sugar and refined grains), low in trans and saturated fats and low in red meat and processed food. A healthy diet should include healthful carbs like fruits, vegetables, whole grains, legumes and soy products. Instead of red meat, turn to fish, like salmon, as a source of protein. A helpful tip to guide yourself to the best food choices at a grocery store is this: Stay around the perimeter of the store. Stay out of the aisles as much as possible.

5.7 Hydrogenated oils are a very bad thing

Hydrogenated oil is made by adding hydrogen to vegetable oil through a process called hydrogenation. The chemical change produces trans fats and makes the oil less likely to spoil, and when used in the manufacturing of foods, helps foods stay fresh longer and have a less greasy feel.

Though research has been extensive, no one is certain why the addition of hydrogen to oil increases a person's cholesterol more than other types of fats do. In fact, trans fat is considered by many to be the worst type of fat. Unlike other fats, trans fat both raises "bad" (LDL) cholesterol and lowers "good" (HDL) cholesterol.

A high LDL cholesterol level in combination with a low HDL cholesterol level increases your risk of heart disease, the leading killer of men and women. Heart disease may lead the tragic list of maladies caused by cholesterol, but it's not the only one.

Hydrogenated oil consumption is also linked to cancer, type 2 diabetes, autoimmune disease and even allergies.

5.8 Looking for a crunch?

Many people experience the need to eat crunchy things. Hence, the popularity of potato chips and other popular dip-bearing crunchies. One of the secrets to creating a healthy diet is to find crunch substitutes.

Celery and carrots are old standbys. For example, in place of crackers, cut carrots on the bias and make crispy carrot rounds. Using a vegetable peeler works well. For some reason, cutting them at a 45-degree angle makes a difference in their crunch!

Instead of croutons, almonds are a healthier alternative for providing a pleasing crunch in salads.

Homemade granola is another great option. On page 60 you'll find a recipe that will knock your socks off.

Homemade Granola Recipe

13 cups of rolled oats	11 cups dried cherries
$1^{1/2}$ cups chopped almonds	1 cup blended flaxseed
1 cup pecans	3 teaspoons hot water
1 cup walnuts	$2^{1/2}$ cups honey
1 cup craisins	$1^{1/2}$ cups canola oil

• Preheat oven to 350 degrees.

• Pour oats, nuts, flaxseed and fruit into a
   very large mixing bowl.

• In another bowl, pour oil, honey, hot water and mix it well.

• Pour the honey mixture over the dry ingredients.
   Mix until they are well coated.

• Pour onto cookie sheets in thin layers.

• Put in oven for seven minutes.

• Take out and toss to make sure granola is not sticking
   to cookie sheets.

• Put in oven for another seven minutes and repeat,
   for a total cooking time of 21 minutes.

• Pour out granola and let dry. If you like it moist,
   put in zipped bags.

5.9

Eat these foods

As with the rest of life, the secret to a healthy diet is eating any food in moderation. That said, some foods are almost always a good go-to food choice. Mix it up. Don't get stuck on any one fruit, vegetable, spice or texture. This is not a comprehensive list, but a list of suggested snacks and ingredients to use to prepare healthy meals.

- ☐ Almonds
- ☐ Apples
- ☐ Apricots
- ☐ Asparagus
- ☐ Avocados
- ☐ Bell peppers
- ☐ Blackberries
- ☐ Blueberries
- ☐ Bok Choy
- ☐ Bran
- ☐ Bran cereal
- ☐ Broccoli
- ☐ Brown rice
- ☐ Brussels sprouts
- ☐ Cabbage
- ☐ Carrots
- ☐ Cauliflower
- ☐ Celery
- ☐ Chard
- ☐ Cloves
- ☐ Cinnamon
- ☐ Collards
- ☐ Cranberries
- ☐ Eggplant
- ☐ Endive
- ☐ Fennel
- ☐ Fish
- ☐ Grapes
- ☐ Green onions
- ☐ Jicama
- ☐ Leeks
- ☐ Lettuce
- ☐ Kale
- ☐ Okra
- ☐ Onions
- ☐ Oranges
- ☐ Melons
- ☐ Mushrooms
- ☐ Mustard greens
- ☐ Peaches
- ☐ Pumpkin seeds
- ☐ Quinoa
- ☐ Radishes
- ☐ Raisins
- ☐ Raspberries
- ☐ Rutabagas
- ☐ Salmon
- ☐ Scallions
- ☐ Snow peas
- ☐ Spaghetti squash
- ☐ Spinach
- ☐ Sprouts
- ☐ Strawberries
- ☐ Tomatoes
- ☐ Tomatilla
- ☐ Tuna
- ☐ Turnips
- ☐ Zucchini

5.10

Color theory

People pay close attention to the color of the clothes they wear, but few people ever consider the hues on their plates at every meal.

When it comes to eating, color is important. Fashionistas will tell you not to wear white shoes after Labor Day. Dietitians will tell you not to eat white food — *ever*.

In the nutrition world, bad carbs like sugar, baked goods made with white flour and other refined carbohydrates are called white food, and they are primary culprits in rising obesity and diabetes rates in the United States. In a nutshell, if it's white and creamy — don't eat it. It is unhealthy and a bad thing for your system.

But not all white food is white food. Natural, unprocessed white food — including onions, cauliflower, turnips and white beans — are not in the same category. These foods are colored by pigments called anthoxanthins and may contain health-promoting chemicals like allicin, which can lower cholesterol and blood pressure and help reduce the risk of heart disease and stomach cancer. Other beneficial white fruits and vegetables include bananas, garlic, ginger, jicama, mushrooms, parsnips and potatoes.

Although carbohydrates are essential, their consumption should be limited to fruits, vegetables, legumes and whole grains. When selecting food for your meals, think of your plate as an artist's palette. Choose a variety of different colors of fruits and vegetables every day.

People who eat more generous amounts of fruits and vegetables are less likely to have chronic diseases, including strokes, type 2 diabetes, some forms of cancer, heart disease and high blood pressure.

Red fruits and vegetables are hued with lycopene or anthocyanins. Lycopene, which is found in tomatoes, watermelon and pink grapefruit, can help reduce the risk of some cancers, including prostate cancer. Anthocyanins can be found in strawberries, raspberries and red grapes. These antioxidants are known to protect cells from damage and have been linked to heart health. Other healthy reds are apples, beets, cabbage, cherries, cranberries, peppers, pomegranates, red potatoes, radishes and rhubarb.

Blue and purple fruits and vegetables also are pigmented by anthocyanins, the antioxidants that protect cells from damage. They also may reduce the risk of heart disease, stroke and cancer. Foods in the blue and purple group include blackberries, blueberries, eggplant, figs, juneberries, plums, prunes, grapes and raisins.

Orange and yellow fruits and vegetables contain carotenoids. Carotenoid-rich foods have been linked to healthy mucous membranes and eyes, plus they also can reduce the risk of certain cancers and heart disease and improve the immune system. Citrus fruits, like oranges, are a good source of vitamin C and folate, a B vitamin that can help reduce the risk of birth defects. Fruits and vegetables in this category also include apples, apricots, butternut squash, cantaloupe, carrots, grapefruit, lemons, mangoes, nectarines, papayas, peaches, pears, peppers, persimmons, pineapple, pumpkin, rutabagas, squash, corn, sweet potatoes, tangerines and tomatoes.

Green is definitely a color that should make other foods envious. Green fruits and vegetables are pigmented by chlorophyll and contain lutein, which is associated with eye health. Lutein-rich food includes spinach and other leafy greens, green peppers, peas, cucumbers, and celery. Broccoli, cauliflower, and cabbage contain a substance called indoles, which may help protect against some forms of cancer. Other beneficial greens include apples, artichokes, asparagus, avocadoes, green beans, Brussels sprouts, grapes, melon, kiwi, limes, green onions and zucchini.

5.11 Keeping it real

What do raspberries really taste like? For children who grow up eating treats with artificial fruit flavoring, a raspberry picked fresh from a bush probably has no flavor correlation to the processed candy labeled *raspberry*. The same is true for bananas, strawberries and grapes. Man cannot imitate the true flavor of nature. Humans also can't replicate the inherent natural benefits of fresh fruits and other foods.

Processed foods are looked at in American culture as conveniences, but in reality, they are more poison than food. Processed ingredients like oils, fats, sugar and sweeteners, flours, starches and salt are depleted of nutrients and provide little nourishment but plenty of empty calories.

The purpose of processing food is to create durable, accessible, attractive, ready-to-eat or ready-to-heat products. Food manufacturers use ultra-processing methods to reduce microbial deterioration to prolong shelf life, to make it possible to transport goods long distance and to make them more enticing and habit-forming.

Processed products are more energy-dense than unprocessed foods and contain oils, solid fats, sugars, salt, flours, and starches that make them excessive in total fat, saturated or trans fat, sugar and sodium — and short of nutrients and dietary fiber.

Chemicals are not nutrients. Even products labeled *light, premium, supplemented* or *fortified* could never be as healthy as fresh fruit or vegetables straight from a farm.

But Americans have become dependent on others for their food. Not only do we purchase what we eat at stores rather than growing it ourselves, we even rely on others to prepare what we consume — therefore taking our knowledge of exactly what we are putting into our bodies out of the equation.

We live in the second generation of Americans who don't actually know how to prepare food, many living off of shelf-stable meal packets and frozen dinners. A survey found that 23 meals a month per household are prepackaged. This number is even higher for adults between the ages of 18 and 34. Restaurants now account for 49 percent of food dollars spent in this country. That number was only 25 percent in 1955. As Americans have lost control of preparing their own food, they also had a rise in obesity and a decline in overall health.

Making wholesome meals for yourself — rich in protein and fresh fruits and vegetables — might seem like an inconvenience, but the simple procedure could add years to your life.

Fast food is a quick path to an early death.

"Eating is an agricultural act."
— *Wendell Berry*

5.12

Eat less, live longer

Reducing your calorie intake may slow the aging process, lessen the chance of heart problems, and reduce the risk of diabetes and other chronic disease.

Calorie restriction, a movement also referred to as "CR," balances calorie reduction with consuming adequate nutrients. People who follow the principle claim that calorie reduction leads to weight loss and a slower metabolic rate, which can actually increase longevity.

Followers generally use 20 to 30 percent as a guideline, cutting their calorie intake by up to 30 percent of the standard recommendation. The plan puts an emphasis on vegetables, fruits and whole grains and frowns upon sugar, fats and most dairy.

A study in the *American Journal of Physiology, Endocrinology and Metabolism* reported interesting findings about CR. In middle-aged adults, calorie restriction led to significant declines in the risks associated with heart disease and heart attacks. Research in Proceedings of the National Academy of Sciences of the United States of America found that people who restricted calories showed lower total and LDL cholesterol, higher HDL cholesterol (the good kind) and lower triglycerides — the fat in the blood stream — than the average American.

"Eat little; sleep sound."
—Iranian Proverb

"Life consists not simply in what
heredity and environment do to us
but in what we make out of
what they do to us. ."
— *Harry Emerson Fosdick*

CHAPTER **6.** Family history

Wellness Wake-up Call

Take a long, hard look at your family history. Ask questions to fill in the gaps. Based on your biological brothers, sisters, parents and grandparents, make a list of the diseases each has had. Chances are high that you have a genetic predisposition for some, or even all, of those ailments. Make sure your lifestyle is not one that will succumb to waking those genetic markers. That's a Wellness Wake-up Call.

6.2

Family tradition

When you flip through a family photo album, do you see your own face reflected in images from the past? Perhaps you have your mother's blue eyes or an uncle's stature. So much of who we are is based on our family heritage.

But our genes define more than just the way we look. Having a close family member with a chronic disease — including cancer, heart disease or diabetes — can increase your risk of developing that disease.

Sit down and make a family tree based on your biological brothers and sisters, parents and grandparents. Next to each name, list any chronic illnesses that have occurred. Denote the age of diagnosis and the age and cause of death of any deceased family members.

Every disease on that list is part of your genetic makeup, and you have an increased chance of being diagnosed with the illness at some point in your life.

According to the Center for Disease Control and Prevention, 96 percent of Americans believe that family history is related to health, but only 30 percent have tried to collect and organize their family health history. What are you waiting for?

Genes play a role in nine of the 10 leading causes of death in the United States, especially cancer and heart disease.

Documenting your family's health is like balancing a checkbook. Although it may bring up some unpleasant realities, it can provide the information you need to stay on target with your own health.

Whether it is breast cancer or stroke, having a predisposition to an illness can give you the knowledge you need to work with your physicians on health maintenance. Your family history provides integral tools for prevention, diagnosis and treatment.

> "Genetics play a huge part in who we are,
> but we also have free will."
> — *Aidan Quinn*

6.3

Fighting the code

Your grandmother was obese, your parents are both overweight and you have gained an extra five pounds every year since you got married. You feel like you can't fight genetics, and you resign yourself to a life of shopping in the plus department. Every time you have to go up a size in jeans, you blame it on your genes.

You are not alone.

Other people feel the same defeat when it comes to chronic illnesses like cancer, diabetes or cardiovascular disease. A genetic predisposition often seems like a ticking time bomb. Although genes do play an important role in our health, scientists are discovering that they are only part of the equation. We actually have more control of our destiny than our family histories would lead us to believe. Although epigenetics may not be a household word, it probably should be. The field of science could be a saving grace for millions of Americans with chronic diseases.

A disease may already be mapped out in your future, but that doesn't mean you can't change paths — and alter the course of your genetics.

"I'm one of those people you hate because of genetics. It's the truth."
— Brad Pitt

6.4   What is epigenetics?

Philosophers will tell you that history repeats itself.

If you look at the history of the world, it seems like humans continue to make the same mistakes over and over. Is it a matter of fate, or do we just make bad choices? Our family health histories are very similar. Although genetics would suggest that chronic illnesses can be fated upon us, an emerging field called epigenetics has discovered evidence that hereditary diseases aren't necessarily a given in people's lives. In fact, knowing your family's personal history can help you write your own future. Predisposition can be circumvented.

Evidently, genes are greatly influenced by their environments. Chemical reactions orchestrate the development and maintenance of an organism, switching parts of the genome off and on at strategic times and locations. Epigenetics is the study of these reactions and why they occur.

In a sense, when it comes to genes, nature versus nurture is at play, and both play a role in an individual's heath.

But epigenetics is important to more than just your own health. Environmental factors and the choices you make not only affect your life, they also have consequences for your children and grandchildren. Choice actually plays a significant role. You are not at the mercy of your genes.

6.5   Darwin was wrong (about some things)

Celebrated 19th-century naturalist Charles Darwin revolutionized the world with his theories about evolution. His observations in 1859's *On the Origin of Species* paved the way for modern science and are the foundation for most of what we know about genetics.

But recent discoveries are showing that Darwin may have missed a few key details. The naturalist believed that genes cannot be affected by the outside world. One of his predecessors, however, had a different viewpoint.

French naturalist Jean-Baptiste Lamarck, who died in 1829, believed that if an organism changes during its lifetime as a form of adaptation to its environment, the changes could be passed along to its offspring.

"In every animal which has not passed the limit of its development, a more frequent and continuous use of any organ gradually strengthens, develops and enlarges that organ, and gives it a power proportional to the length of time it has been so used; while the permanent disuse of any organ imperceptibly weakens and deteriorates it, and progressively diminishes its functional capacity, until it finally disappears," LaMarck wrote in 1809 in *Philosophie Zoologique*.

Recent research has shown that LaMarck's theory of environmental influences on genetics, which was discredited in the 19th century, actually has validity.

Epigenetic research has found that genes are only 15 percent of the total genetic material you get from your parents. The epigenome, which accounts for the remaining 85 percent, is a scaffolding of proteins that surrounds the DNA double-helix pattern. The scaffolding works as an interface and interacts with your environment.

The epigenome, responding to lifestyle choices, can turn the genes on or off, which changes the way your body translates your genetic coding.

Conscious decisions to improve your health actually can interact with your epigenome. The proteins in your epigenome can react to your choices and turn off genes that otherwise might have expressed themselves as disease in former generations.

While epigenetics can have beneficial implications for you, it also can have dire repercussions for your descendants. Just as your epigenome can be altered by your lifestyle choices, the negative lifestyle choices you make can alter the epigenome passed on to your children and grandchildren.

In other words, the choices you make are important for both your own health and the health of subsequent generations.

"Genetics were kind, but I work very hard."
— *Anna Paquin*

6.6

Of mice and men

All mice are not created equal.

To aid scientists, research suppliers have warehouses filled with thousands of mice, all specifically bred to have certain genetic defects.

The agouti mouse is bred to be obese with yellow fur, instead of the normal brown. The rodents are predisposed to heart disease, diabetes and cancer.

In a Duke University study, researchers fed agouti mice a diet that contained additives of folic acid, vitamin B12 and chlorine, nutrients meant to increase methylation of the protein coat around the DNA. The mice were then put into breeding situations.

The mice that had received the supplements all gave birth to normal offspring, complete with brown coats and of a healthy weight. The agouti gene remained part of their DNA, but it was not expressed in the offspring.

The diet silenced the bad genes in the agouti mothers, and their lifestyle choices had a positive effect on the next generation. Similarly, when pregnant agouti mice ingested BPA, a compound commonly used to make polycarbonate plastic water bottles, a larger number of their babies were born yellow and unhealthy. The exposure to BPA during their early development had caused decreased methylation of the agouti gene. Conversely, when the BPA-exposed mothers were fed methyl-rich foods, the offspring were predominantly brown and healthy.

Male rats deprived of food before mating produce offspring with less blood sugar and altered levels of corticosterone, which protects against stress, and an insulin-like growth factor that helps babies develop. But diet isn't the only environmental factor documented to have an effect on epigenetics in rodents. Researchers have found that a rat mother's nurturing of her young can affect how the pups react to stress later in life. When the female children reach adulthood and become mothers, the ones that received high-quality care become high-nurturing mothers. The pups who received low-quality care become poor nurturers.

Another study placed small field mice in cages with large, aggressive males. The larger rodents were allowed to attack and bully the field mice for about five minutes a day for 10 days. By the end of the period, about two-thirds of the field mice had signs of permanent depression, anxiety and post-traumatic stress disorder.

The field mice were bred with normal females. When their pups grew up, they too showed signs of depression and anxiety, avoiding other mice whenever possible.

Epigenetic marks can be passed from parent to offspring in a way that completely bypasses egg or sperm. Parental behavior can transmit epigenetic information onto their offspring's DNA.

6.7   One of these things isn't like the other

To prove that genetics isn't always a finite predictor of health, a number of scientists are looking at identical twins. Identical twins develop from a single zygote and have the same genome. So in theory, they should be exact copies of one another. For more than a century, researchers have been looking at twins as the perfect case study for a genetic showdown of nature versus nurture.

Twins are an ideal model for examining how environment and genes interact. Although identical twins certainly look alike and may share many personal traits — including eye color and facial features — they are far from identical. Consider the fact that it is not uncommon for one twin to develop a chronic disease, while the other sibling remains healthy. But if twins develop from a single zygote, shouldn't they both develop the same illnesses at roughly the same time?

If disease were purely a factor of DNA, then yes. But obviously another force is at play. Environmental factors can alter our genetics. In fact, epigenetics is almost like a bridge between our genes and our environment.

Scientists have observed that as twins age, epigenetic differences begin to take place, especially when the individuals make different lifestyle choices. If one twin has bad dietary habits, smokes or drinks, those behaviors could affect the epigenomes in a negative way.

When monozygotic twins have different diseases at different times, scientists call the phenomenon twin discordance.

In a groundbreaking study published in *Genome Research*, scientists in the United States and Spain analyzed sets of twins where one had developed the autoimmune disease lupus. The results show that environmental factors, such as diet and chemical exposure, definitely have an influence on epigenomes.

"Our study suggests that the effect of the environment or differences in lifestyle may leave a molecular mark in key genes for immune function that contributes to the differential onset of the disease in twins," said Dr. Esteban Ballestar, senior author of the study.

Cancer researchers have found similar information in pairs of identical twins.

As the chemical tags that control genes change, cells can become abnormal, even triggering disease like cancer. While cancer traditionally has been viewed as a disease resulting from broken genes, the reality is that epigenomes also come into play.

Twin research has shown that having a genetic predisposition to cancer and other illnesses doesn't necessarily mean that a person will get the disease. Lifestyle choices are a key factor in how the genes react.

> "I got a hundred bucks says my baby beats
> Pete's baby. I think genetics are in my favor."
> — *Andre Agassi*

6.8 Epigenomes know best

Mothers aren't the only parents passing on epigenetic traits to their offspring.

Fathers are equally important in the health equation, as showcased in some of the rodent research previously mentioned. Pregnant women are taught to be cautious of everything from smoking to the foods they eat, but a father's behavior can be just as detrimental. In fact, lifestyle choices a man makes even years before conception can be reflected in his epigenetics and passed on to his children.

Overkalix, a village in the corner of northern Sweden, documents the powerful effect nutrition has on the genetic material fathers pass on to their children. Until the 20th century, Overkalix was unreachable by road or train. When the village had bad agricultural harvests, the children starved. When crops were good, people ate more than they needed.

Looking at figures going back as far as 1799, researchers correlated children's health data with records of regional harvests. The findings divulged some interesting points about epigenetics.

Males who had poor nutrition during the years right before puberty ended up having sons who, as adults, had lower than normal rates of heart disease. Boys who had consumed too much food during the ages of 9 to 12 had grandsons with a higher rate of diabetes.

The prepubescent diet permanently reprogrammed the epigenetic switches that controlled the development of sperm years later. Those reprogrammed switches seemed to be transferred to sons and grandsons.

A father's age at the time of conception also could have epigenetic effects on his offspring.

A 40-year-old man's gonad cells have divided 610 times to make spermatozoa, whereas a woman is born with all the eggs she will every carry. That number goes up to 840 by the time a man is in his 50s. The more times cells copy themselves, the more likely it is that mistakes will appear in the DNA chain. Some researchers even speculate that a percentage of the mistakes are based on environmental epigenetic markings, which can affect brain development.

As more and more research is being done on mental disorders, scientists are seeing indications that children of older fathers show more signs of autism, schizophrenia and bipolar disorder than children of younger men.

Men's life experiences leave biological traces on their children and grandchildren. Everything from the food men eat to the toxins they absorb — and even traumas they may endure — can be passed on to future generations through epigenetics.

"I am very comfortable with the fact that
we can override biology with free will."
— *Richard Dawkins*

6.9 Practical terms

Your future is about more than just your genes.

Science is showing that the way you interact with your genes through diet, lifestyle, and the environment will be the real indicator of your lifespan.

You can change how your genes are expressed.

The genes in your body that can't be changed are less than 2 percent. That means that 98 percent of your genetic material can be modified and turned on or off.

Every choice you make has some influence on your epigenetics — and the epigenetics of your children and your children's children.

A diet of fast food and sugar soda will expand your waistline and affect your health, but it also will predispose future generations to chronic illnesses like heart disease, diabetes, and obesity.

It's important to know your family's health history, but genetics is only part of the discussion.

The foods we eat, the chemicals we consume and breathe, our level of activity and even our social environment can actually alter our genes.

You can fight genetics; you just have to use the right weapons.

"'Tis healthy to be sick sometimes."
— Henry David Thoreau

CHAPTER 7. Immune system

Wellness Wake-up Call

How many times in the last year have you or a family member missed work? How many times do you go to the doctor and get antibiotics? Or, next time you take your child to the pediatrician, ask the nurse to review the file and see how many times your child has been on antibiotics. If you or others in your family get sick multiple times a year — or at the same time every year, that's a Wellness Wake-up Call.

7.2

Supporting players

Most people take their health for granted. While we are healthy, we rarely consider the intricate network of defense our body naturally has to protect us from disease. Even operating while we sleep, our bodies' natural protectors are on constant guard from invaders.

The immune system and lymphatic system are like supporting actors who steal every scene in a movie. Although we don't think about them often, they are always hard at work. The show couldn't go on without them, and our bodies owe every successful performance to their efforts behind the scenes.

Think of your body as a football stadium. The home team, which is made up of the immune and lymphatic systems, is in a fierce battle against the visiting team, which is made up mostly of viruses and bacteria. Much like in football, sometimes the best offense is a good defense — and the immune system deserves to win an MVP award every season. Drawing from its own history, it faces every opponent with a complex strategy that requires strength, numbers and teamwork. In the game of life, the immune system is willing to fight to the death.

Our organs, tissue, cells and cell products naturally protect us from substances that enter the body from the environment. Even our skin and mucous membranes play an important role by creating a barrier to prevent millions of organisms from breaking through the fortress.

When a foreign substance does manage to get past these anatomic barriers, the body responds with its next defense — inflammation.

Inflammation is like an attack. The body is trying to excrete the invaders, and its strategies include sneezing, runny noses and fever. These symptoms might make us feel uncomfortable, but they are actually signs that the body is fighting illness. The next time you sneeze, just try to think of it as a tactical response to a foreign invasion.

Some viruses and bacteria are more virulent. When the inflammation defense fails to rid the body of invaders, the immune system kicks in and takes over. White blood cells go after the infection and attack antigens, which could be any foreign substance — from a virus to a sliver. A healthy adult has up to 25,000 white blood cells in a single drop of blood. Lymphocytes, which account for about a quarter of all white blood cells, travel to the lymph nodes, part of the lymphatic system, and aid in battling disease.

There are two main fluids in the body — blood and lymph. Both help distribute our body's natural defenses throughout the other systems. The lymphatic system works with the immune system to filter out organisms that cause disease and generate antibodies. The primary lymphoid organs are the thymus and bone marrow, but the system also includes lymph nodes, tonsils, the spleen and Peyer's patches in the intestinal wall. Made up of a network of vessels that help circulate body fluids and white blood cells, the system distributes nutrients and fluids and also drains excess fluids so tissues in the body do not swell.

Centuries ago, physicians realized the power of the immune system when they noticed that people who had recovered from the plague never got the often fatal disease again. They had acquired an immunity to the bacterial infection. Our immune system, with a little help from the lymphatic system, has an excellent memory. Once it has conquered a virus, it develops the perfect strategy for any future attacks.

> "Understanding the laws of nature does not mean that we are immune to their operations."
> — *David Gerrold*

7.3   Hard pill to swallow

Around 61 percent of adults regularly use at least one drug to treat their health problems, and that number has risen nearly 15 percent in a decade. As we age, the numbers get even higher. More than 25 percent of seniors take at least five different medications on a daily basis.

According to Sophia De Monte, a spokeswoman for the American Pharmacists Association, multiple prescriptions taken at once can have serious consequences.

"As you keep increasing the amount of prescriptions, that increases the chance of having a drug interaction or major side effect," De Monte said. "It's exponential. The more you add on, the more chance you'll have something bad happen."

The average American is prescribed medication about 13 times a year, according to a report from the Kaiser Family Foundation. Our country has become a culture reliant on pills. Instead of focusing on overall health and wellness, we look for a magic and instant cure for everything that ails us. We would rather medicate ourselves than eat properly and exercise. Unfortunately, the answer to all of our problems can't be found in a bottle.

Take the common cold or flu for example. Most people are actually better off allowing the virus to run its course, according to Dr. Ben Kim, a proponent of natural health care. Bed rest is the best treatment, and over-the-counter drugs that suppress the symptoms may actually extend the length of the illness.

Kim points out that the viruses that cause colds and flu mainly infect the body's weakest cells, which already are burdened with excessive waste products and toxins. By getting rid of these cells, the body is able to produce healthy replacements. "Have you ever been amazed by how much 'stuff' you could blow out of your nose while you had a cold or a flu? Embedded within all of that mucous are countless dead cells that your body is saying goodbye to, largely due to the effect of viruses," Kim writes.

By suppressing symptoms, like a runny nose and cough, over-the-counter medications make it more difficult for the body to complete the cleansing process. Although you might not feel as uncomfortable, your body will take longer to heal.

Even worse, many physicians will prescribe antibiotics to patients with cold and flu symptoms. Antibiotics will kill a bacterial infection, but they do nothing against viruses. According to the *Prescriber's Newsletter*, a common medical reference, only 1 in 4,000 patients with cold symptoms will actually have a serious sickness that can be helped by a physician's prescription. Yet, a study published in the *Journal of the American Medical Association* showed that doctors prescribed antibiotics for more than 60 percent of adults with upper respiratory tract infections, which are usually the result of a virus.

"People who take antibiotics while suffering with a cold or flu often feel slightly better because antibiotics have a mild anti-inflammatory effect," Kim explained.

"But this benefit is far outweighed by the negative impact that antibiotics have on friendly bacteria that live throughout your digestive tract."

The good bacteria in our intestines help make vitamins and boost immunity. Killing them off with antibiotics may be contributing to the increase in chronic health conditions, including obesity, asthma and cancer. But the extinction of bacteria in the intestine is more than just a hypothesis. Dr. Martin Blaser, head of the department of medicine at New York University's Langone Medical Center, has seen evidence that H. pylori, an intestinal bacterium that was once common, is on its way to extinction. Less than 100 years ago, it was the main microbe present in the human stomach. Yet today, less than 6 percent of children born in the United States, Sweden and Germany have the organism. Although the health consequences are unclear, the eradication suggests, according to Blaser, that other stomach and intestinal bacteria also are becoming dinosaurs.

Since Alexander Fleming first discovered penicillin in 1927, antibiotics have transformed medical care. But the prevalent use of antibiotics has had a cost. According to the Centers for Disease Control and Prevention, antibiotic resistance is one of the world's most pressing public health issues. Drug-resistant superbugs could become a real global threat.

"The deviation of man from the state in which he was originally placed by nature seems to have proved to him a prolific source of diseases."
— *Edward Jenner*

7.4 A little dirty talk

Americans have become obsessed with cleanliness. Television commercials teach us that germs are lurking on every surface of our homes and prod us to find chemical solutions to these frightening intruders. We're encouraged to spray, wipe and scrub our concerns away. Antimicrobial soaps and hand sanitizers make promises of better health, and 75 percent of American households now use the products. Even common objects like chopping boards, refrigerators, lunch boxes and mattresses are being treated with triclosan and triclocarban, compounds prevalent in antibiotic wipes. But our focus on sanitation might actually be bad for us, according to a growing field of research.

"Our immune system was built for more action than it gets," said Dr. Jordan S. Orange, chief of immunology, allergy and rheumatology at Texas Children's Hospital. "We were once born into piles of dirt. Our immune systems have evolved to handle these challenges extremely well. But, in our modern society, it's not something we're up against that much."

Viruses, however, are continually battling our antibiotic world, and they are getting stronger. The organisms learn to adapt and mutate. "Dousing everything we touch with antibacterial soaps and taking antibiotic medications at the first sign of a cold can upset the natural balance of microorganisms in and around us, leaving behind only the 'superbugs,'" said Dr. Stuart Levy, a microbiologist at Tufts University.

Levy is one of many scientists who believe in "The Hygiene Hypothesis," a theory that our recent obsession with fighting germs is actually causing us more harm than good. For example, children who are not exposed to a wide variety of bacteria may have immune systems that overreact to pollen and dust or become allergic to otherwise harmless substances. It also might explain the recent rise in autoimmune disorders.

"Just as a child needs lots of exercise to develop strong bones and muscles, a child's immune system needs a rigorous workout to develop normal resistance to infections throughout life," Levy said.

Although Americans have been convinced by million-dollar marketing campaigns that antibiotic soap is healthier, research data shows otherwise. Allison Aiello, a professor at the University of Michigan analyzed a number of studies on the effectiveness of hand-washing strategies. According to her findings, antibiotic soaps and wipes with triclosan were no more likely than regular soap to prevent gastrointestinal or respiratory infections.

In one study conducted in Pakistan, gastrointestinal illnesses were reduced by half when people washed their hands with basic soap. They were reduced by a little less than half when they used antibiotic soap.

A Columbia University research project had even worse results. Although statistics showed no difference between the effects of the two for healthy hand washers, chronically sick patients actually had an increase in the frequency of fevers, runny noses and coughs when they washed with antibiotic soap. The real key to staying healthy is not using antimicrobial products, it's washing your hands. Scientists estimate that proper hand washing with regular soap can reduce the frequency that people get sick by as much as 40 percent.

But if you are looking for scary facts, here's something that should really keep you up at night worried about germs. Few people actually take hygiene seriously. In a study of nearly 8,000 people in five American cities, around 50 percent of the participants didn't wash their hands after going to the bathroom.

> "I was naseous and tingly all over.
> I was either in love or I had smallpox"
> — *Woody Allen*

7.5 Food for thought

A cow isn't necessarily a cow and a chicken might not even resemble the feathered creatures that roamed barnyards 100 years ago. Through the use of chemicals, antibiotics and hormones, farming has become more industrial than natural.

"Modern production of foods incorporates a wide range of synthetic chemicals," said Jeff Gillman, author of *The Truth About Organic Gardening*. "Many of these chemicals have the potential to be very damaging to humans if they are exposed to high concentrations, or to low concentrations over an extended period of time."

Although additives to food are monitored by government agencies, a wave of natural food proponents is skeptical about the standards being applied.

"More people are realizing that there is a myriad of chemicals in conventionally produced food," said Craig Minowa, an environmental scientist with the Organic Consumers Association.

Each chemical has to pass a safety review, but no one monitors what they may do when used in combinations. Just as there can be a cumulative negative effect when people take multiple drug prescriptions at the same time, food additives could have similar negative consequences.

When you purchase a steak at the supermarket, do you know what you're really buying for the backyard barbecue? In addition to a cut of meat, you might be consuming a slew of antibiotics.

Many cattle producers feed antibiotics in a low dose on a daily base to their livestock. The medication isn't to prevent them from getting sick, it's to make them gain weight. Companies aren't required to label meat or provide information about whether it contains antibiotics, so there's no way to be certain if the steak you are purchasing at the grocery store is filled with antibiotics.

According to the *New England Journal of Medicine*, 20 percent of ground beef sold at supermarkets contains salmonella — and of that amount, 84 percent contains a Salmonella bacterium that is resistant to some antibiotics. Similarly, researchers have been able to link resistant strains of Salmonella to pork from pigs fed the antibiotic ciprofloxacin. The Food and Drug Administration also estimates that within a single year, chickens that had been given antibiotics directly caused 11,000 people to catch intestinal illnesses from antibiotic-resistance bacteria.

But just how prevalent are antibiotics in food? About 80 percent of the antibiotics sold in the United States — and this statistic takes into account the frequent prescriptions given by physicians — goes to chickens, cows, pigs and other animals that people eat. Despite this staggering percentage, food producers are not required to report how they use the drugs they purchase — not even the quantities they administer to a single animal.

As far back as 1977, the FDA announced that it had plans to ban the use of antibiotics in some agricultural products. Because it would have hurt the big-business profits of corporate farming, companies with a lot of money and influence fought back. The House and Senate quickly passed resolutions against any bans, and the FDA stepped back from its stance.

As animals continue to be treated with antibiotics, over time, the bacteria living in those animals will become resistant to the drugs. Humans who consume those animals and are exposed to resistant bacteria because of improperly cooked or prepared meat won't respond to antibiotic treatment.

"The single biggest problem we face in infectious disease today is the rapid growth of resistance to antibiotics," said Glenn Morris, director of the Emerging Pathogens Institute at the University of Florida. "Human use contributes to that, but use in animals clearly has a part, too."

The World Health Organization has addressed the issue and called for a reduction in the overuse of antimicrobials in food animals. The group recommends that prescriptions be required for all antibiotics used to treat sick animals and urges the termination of antibiotics used for growth promotion by food producers.

"The first wealth is health"
— *Ralph Waldo Emerson*

7.6   Shot in the arm

Modern Americans want a quick fix. We want to believe that pain and suffering are outdated. We want life to be perfect, and we put our faith in science. People view health as an entitlement, and we expect doctors to keep us well with magic pills and shots. Sickness is not part of the plan.

People in the 21st century want to believe that scientists can create vaccines to prevent every little ache and pain. We expect to be invincible. But humans weren't meant to be ensconced in a bubble-wrapped layer of protection from the outside world. We co-exist in an environment filled with bacteria and viruses — some more dangerous than others. By constantly trying to avoid these germs in our lives, humans are becoming fragile — and the bacteria and viruses are getting stronger.

The word *epidemic* sends shivers up our spines. Hollywood has fueled our fear of disease with blockbuster films like *Outbreak* and *Contagion*. Even the recent pop culture zombie phenomenon is linked to our anxiety about bacteria, viruses and the threat of a pandemic — a widespread health crisis.

Unlike vampires and other movie monsters, viruses are real and history has shown us just how scary they can be. In 14th-century Europe, the Black Death, a bacterial plague, killed nearly 200 million people in a little more than a decade.

Yellow fever, an acute viral infection spread through mosquito bites, killed more than 41,000 people in New Orleans, a community hard hit because of its tropical climate, between the years of 1817 and 1905, the city's last epidemic. More recently, AIDS, a disease caused by a viral infection that attacks the immune system, has killed more than 600,000 people in the United States alone since it was first discovered in 1981.

These staggering statistics are enough to scare anyone. If a shot could have prevented even a fraction of these deaths, most people would jump at the opportunity to promote its development. Vaccines seem like a sure-fire way to protect us from the horrors of the world. Poliomyelitis, better known as polio, caused a fear as frightening as the Red Scare in America in the 1950s. The disease, which can attack the central nervous system, crippled thousands of people, primarily young children. In 1955, Jonas Salk, a researcher at the University of Pittsburgh, was seen as a savior for his development of a polio vaccine.

Today, polio seems like a ghost of the past, much like the Black Death and Yellow Fever. Because we see few examples of the disease in our time, we feel like the vaccine was a miracle cure. Natural immunity and vaccine-induced immunity are very different. Many disease-causing organisms enter our bodies through the mucous membranes of the mouth, nose, pulmonary system or digestive tract. The mucous membranes have their own immune response, which is the body's first line of defense. Our bodies naturally fight off invading organisms at these entry points, often reducing or even eliminating the need for the immune system to kick into activation. As soon as children are born, they begin to develop natural immunity to thousands of microorganisms. Every time they eat, breathe or touch their skin they are exposed to something new — and it makes them stronger. The immune systems built in the linings of places like the nose and throat develop a history to protect the body from invaders.

Vaccines create an antibody, but they do not impart long-term immunity. The body's own defense mechanisms do not create the same kind of memory that occurs when you breathe, eat or are exposed to a virus or bacteria through the skin.

"The attempt to eradicate entire microbial species from the biosphere must inevitably upset the balance of Nature in fundamental ways that we can barely imagine," writes Dr. Richard Moskowitz. "Such concerns loom ever larger as new vaccines continue to be developed for no better reason than that we have the technical capacity to make them — and to manipulate the evolutionary process itself."

7.7

A dose of reality

During a period of two years, the average American baby gets 24 shots. In a single visit to the doctor, a child can get as many as five inoculations. Children are seen as fragile little creatures that we want to protect from every danger. From pertussis to diphtheria and tetanus shots (DTaP), immunization has become a standard part of early child care in our country. More than 77 percent of kids on their first day of school are completely up-to-date on the regimen of shots.

We trust our doctors, and we believe these vaccinations are keeping them safe. But a growing number of parents and medical professionals are starting to question the vaccines that have become a norm in our culture.

According to the American Lung Association, more than 20 million Americans have asthma, including 6.1 million children. Some research studies have linked the increasing incidence of asthma in children to the pertussis, or whooping cough, vaccine. The shot, they speculate, might change the balance of immunity toward allergic responses.

One English study, which followed 1,934 patients from birth to age 12, found that children given a whole-cell vaccine for pertussis were 40 percent more likely to develop asthma than unvaccinated children.

A report from the Centers for Disease Control and Prevention mentions a link between vaccinations for Hib, which protects against a potentially serious influenza, and hepatitis B, which is primarily spread through unprotected sex and intravenous drug use (not a serious risk for infants). "In our main analysis, we found that Hib and hepatitis B vaccines were associated with 10 and 20 percent increases in asthma risk, respectively," the report states.

Although the CDC continues to encourage vaccinations, it does add a cautionary note. "The risk of vaccine-induced asthma could be decreased dramatically by no longer administering a routine hepatitis B vaccine for all newborns, only giving the more necessary vaccines, such as Hib and DTaP, in the first year, and by delaying the first vaccine until after 4 months," the health organization said in a statement.

Are children being vaccinated for comfort rather than maximum health benefits?

For example, Moskowitz points out that measles, although unpleasant, is rarely a life-threatening illness. The symptoms we correlate with the sickness — mainly sneezing and coughing — are actually the body's natural attempt to rid itself of the virus. "For not only will children who recover from the measles never again be susceptible to it; such an experience must also prepare them to respond even more promptly and effectively to whatever other infections they may acquire in the future. Indeed, the ability to mount a vigorous, acute response to organisms of this type must be reckoned among the fundamental requirements of general health and well-being."

A relatively new vaccine for chickenpox, another common childhood illness, also creates some interesting questions. Although the virus strikes many people, it only causes serious complications in less than 1 in 10,000 children.

Dr. Richard Halvorsen, author of *The Truth About Vaccines,* believes the benefits of a shot aren't worth the risks. "We are in danger of becoming dependent on immunization, rather than on our own immune systems, for our future health," he said.

Halvorsen surmises that the chickenpox vaccine could push the disease into older age brackets, who have had the vaccine wear off and will suffer greater symptoms. In addition, he also believes the vaccination is likely to increase the number of people getting shingles, which is caused by the same virus and can have painful and more serious manifestations.

In his statements regarding immunization, Moskowitz finds that people have a blind faith in inoculations. "It is dangerously misleading and indeed the exact opposite of the truth to claim that a vaccine makes us 'immune' or protects us against an acute disease, if in fact it only drives the infection deeper into the interior and causes us to harbor it chronically, with the result that our responses to it become weaker and weaker, and show less and less tendency to heal or resolve themselves spontaneously," he said.

The physician believes our bodies' natural defenses are greater than we want to believe. Humans should put as much faith in nature as they do in science.

"We prefer to forget the older and simpler but more difficult truths, that the susceptibility to illness is deeply rooted in our biological nature, and that the signs and symptoms of disease are the attempt of our own life energy to overcome whatever we are trying to overcome, trying, in short, to heal ourselves."

Science, Halvorsen argues, isn't a replacement for nature. "We are introducing vaccines too readily and without regard to the long-term consequences," he said. "There has been a huge rise over recent years in immune-related diseases, such as diabetes, asthma and eczema; the possible link to vaccines, though controversial, is plausible."

7.8 Fight for rights

Although most school systems have immunization requirements, parents have more options than they may believe. Although inoculation has become a standard in America, it still can be a choice — one that parents should make armed with knowledge.

Physicians can issue waivers for children who have compromised immune systems. In addition, almost every state allows waivers for parents who don't want their children to be immunized because of religious beliefs. A growing number of parents are choosing not to have their children immunized, either entirely or for specific inoculations, and a number of states are passing legislation to protect them. In 20 states, parents are allowed to opt out of required immunizations based on philosophical grounds.

Most children in the United States are immunized, but the numbers are changing. Nearly one-half of 1 percent of children enrolled in schools has a medical waiver for vaccination, and 2 to 3 percent have a non-medical waiver.

Editor's Note: *To be clear, the author advocates that parents give serious thought and consideration to their children's vaccination plan. However, he is not advocating a complete abandonment of vaccinations. Parents should educate themselves and make informed decisions as opposed to following the general rule of thought.*

"Health is the state about which
medicine has nothing to say."
— *W. H. Auden*

7.9

On Mother's Day, we thank mom for all the wonderful things she has brought into our lives. Hallmark makes greeting cards that praise her patience and nurturing, but the company should consider adding immunity to the list of things children can attribute to the matriarch of their family.

Children can link their health not only to their mother's genetics but also to the nourishment she provided during nursing. Breastfeeding is nature's own inoculation to many bacteria and viruses, according to recent research. Human breastmilk provides protective factors against infectious disease and may actually influence immune system development.

Researchers from the West Virginia School of Osteopathic Medicine have found that breastfeeding can protect infants against extraintestinal infections and respiratory diseases. The research also indicates that the process can influence immune development, which can prevent autoimmune disorders, including atopic allergies. In the big picture, nursing might even be linked to the prevention of chronic disease later in life. Breastmilk contains antibodies developed as a consequence of a mother's previous exposures to infection agents. The scientists suggest that these antibodies can bond to potential pathogens and prevent their attachment to an infant's cells.

A joint study between Brigham Young University, Harvard and Stanford identified a molecule that is the key to a mother's ability to pass along an immunity to intestinal infections through her breast milk.

Before a woman is pregnant, the cells that produce antibodies against intestinal infections travel around the circulatory system and end up in the intestine, where they defend against infections like cholera and rotavirus. When a woman begins to lactate, these defenders take a different strategy. Some of the antibody-producing cells head to the mammary glands. When the baby nurses, the antibodies go to the child's intestine and continue the fight against infections originally developed for the mother.

The process also goes the other way. As a baby is exposed to germs, it can be transferred back to the mother during feeding. The mother's body will make antibodies and then transfer them back to the child for protection. According to the researchers, the process explains why formula-fed infants have twice the incidence of diarrhea as babies who are nursed with breast milk. Babies fed with formula also have higher rates of middle ear infections, pneumonia, stomach flu, urinary tract infections and necrotizing enterocolitis, a digestive disorder that is a leading killer of premature infants.

Breastfeeding gives infants added protection against heart disease, immune system cancers like lymphoma, bowel diseases, juvenile rheumatoid arthritis, asthma and allergies, respiratory infections, eczema and type 1 and type 2 diabetes. Breast milk even contains a protein that could reduce the chance of obesity later in life by affecting the way the body processes fat.

Doctors recommend breastfeeding for the first six months after birth, and then mothers should continue to breastfeed with the addition of solid foods for at least six more months.

But breastfeeding isn't just good for children, it also has positive results for mothers. A number of research studies have shown that women who breastfeed have a reduced risk of breast and ovarian cancers and osteoporosis later in life.

"Health is not valued 'til sickness comes."
— *Thomas Fuller*

7.10   Natural immunity

As adults, we have more control over our immune systems than we realize. We don't have to rely on vaccines or antibiotics to keep us well. Maintaining a healthy lifestyle is more important than anything a doctor can do for you. The goal is to prevent disease, not fight it.

It's never too late to give your immune system a boost. Even if you have suffered from disease or chronic illness in the past, what you begin to do today will have a significant role in your future health. Here are 10 tips to help your immune system work more efficiently.

1 Avoid cigarette smoke.

If you smoke cigarettes, stop. If you know people who smoke, ask them to not smoke around you. Cigarette smoke contains more than 4,000 chemical compounds — and at least 43 of them are known carcinogens. Smoking has been linked to heart disease, lung and esophageal cancer and chronic lung disease. But did you know that it also contributes to cancer of the bladder, pancreas and kidneys? Smoking actually kills more than two times as many people as AIDS, alcohol abuse, motor vehicle accidents, homicides, drugs and suicide combined — one of out every five deaths in this country is smoking-related. But the secondhand smoke you inhale can be just as deadly. An estimated 3,000 nonsmoking Americans die of lung cancer each year.

2 Live a life without chemicals.

In modern society, it's hard to avoid all chemicals, but the more you try to delete them from your daily life, the better. Look for natural cleaning products for your home, read food packages carefully, shy away from pesticides, and choose paper goods and households items that are made with less toxic material.

3 Get more sleep.

Sleep deprivation can be a major drain on your immune system. A lack of sleep can reduce your white blood cell count, and research has linked chronic sleep deprivation to heart disease, gastrointestinal problems and other illnesses. In addition to causing bags and dark circles under the eyes, lack of sleep over time has been attributed to premature aging in at least one scientific study.

4 Chill out.

Living a high-stress, Type A-personality lifestyle puts a real damper on the immune system. A number of studies have linked higher levels of stress hormones to rapid cancer progression, and people who are stressed are more prone to cardiovascular disease. Stress lowers white blood cell counts, which can open your body up to a wide range of illnesses.

Let a smile be your umbrella.

Although having a "glass half full" attitude can be difficult at times, maintaining a positive outlook on life is a natural immunity booster. Optimists have a longer life expectancy than pessimists and also have overall better health. A poor outlook and bad mood actually can make you more susceptible to the common cold and flu.

Get up and move.

Being a couch potato is bad for your overall health, but it also affects your immune system. Exercise can help fight high blood pressure, coronary heart disease and type 2 diabetes. Moderate exercise also promotes white blood cells to pulse through the bloodstream, where they can attack antigens sooner.

Make new friends...

— and stay in touch with old ones. Social interaction is crucial to remaining healthy, a number of research reports have found. Researchers who monitored 276 people between the ages of 18 and 55 found interesting results. People who had six or more social connections were four times better at fighting off viruses, especially the ones that cause the common cold.

Laugh a little.

Positive emotions decrease stress hormones and increase immune cells. A California study reported that 10 healthy men who watched a comedy video for an hour showed a significant increase in immune hormones in their systems.

Limit your medications, especially antibiotics.

Only take antibiotics for bacterial infections, and make sure you follow the directions and take the entire course. Never use antibiotics to try to prevent getting an infection, and don't save or share your prescriptions.

Skip processed and packaged food as much as possible.

It's not just what is added to the food that you have to worry about, either. Processed foods are often stripped of healthy nutrients. A poor diet is estimated to kill up to 580,000 Americans each year. Malnourishment weakens the immune system and makes it more difficult to fight disease. Cut your fat take, and decrease your sugar consumption. Sugar inhibits phagocytosis, a process where white blood cells engulf and consume viruses and bacteria.

> "Medicine is the means by which
> we poor feeble creatures try to
> keep from dying or aching."
> — *P. T. Barnum*

7.11   Eat for immunity

The food we eat fuels our bodies. It also can fuel our immune systems. While consuming fat-laden, processed food does little for our overall nutrition, it also weakens our ability to ward off viruses and kill bacteria. Rather than rely on a vaccine to give your white blood cell count a boost, consider changing your diet. Here are 10 things you can buy today to help give your immune system a kick start:

1 **Yogurt.**
Look for packages with a "live and active cultures" seal, which ensures the product has probiotics, healthy bacteria that are good for the digestive tract. An Austrian study from the University of Vienna found that a daily 7-ounce serving of yogurt was as effective as taking medication to help improve immunity.

2 **Garlic.**
The "stinking rose" does more than just ward off vampires. Garlic contains allicin, an active ingredient that fights off infection and bacteria. Studies suggest that people who eat more than six cloves a week have a 30 percent lower rate of colorectal cancer and a 50 percent lower rate of stomach cancer — plus it's good for preventing the common cold. Raw cloves are more effective than cooked ones.

3 **Fish.**
Selenium — which is plentiful in oysters, lobsters, crabs and clams — helps white blood cells produce proteins that clear flu viruses from the body. You can help reduce inflammation, increase your body's airflow and protect yourself from respiratory infections by consuming salmon, mackerel and herring, which are rich in omega-3 fats.

4 Tea.
Both black and green tea (even decaffeinated) have the amino acid L-theanine, a great immune booster. According to a Harvard study, people who drank five cups a day of black tea during a two-week period had 10 times more virus-fighting interferon in their blood.

5 Sweet potatoes.
Skip the brown sugar and marshmallows and let these tubers, which are great for the skin, shine on their own. These vegetables are rich in vitamin A, which plays a role in the production of connective tissue. A half-cup serving delivers 40 percent of the daily recommended amount of the vitamin and only has 170 calories.

6 Mushrooms.
This fungi increases the production and activity of white blood cells, making them more aggressive. Any mushrooms are beneficial, including the common button mushroom, which has both selenium and antioxidants. Animal studies have shown that mushrooms have antiviral, antibacterial and antitumor effects.

7 Almonds.
A ¼-cup serving has nearly 50 percent of the daily recommended amount of Vitamin E, a great immune booster. They also are rich in riboflavin and niacin, B vitamins that are effective in stress relief.

8 Spinach.
Popeye the Sailor was on to something — although he should have chosen fresh over canned. Spinach is a "super" food that contains folate, which helps the body produce new cells and repair DNA. Eat it raw or lightly cooked for the best benefits.

9 Cabbage.
The leafy vegetable is a great source of glutamine and it also is rich in antioxidants. White, red or Chinese cabbages all contain beneficial nutrients.

10 Broccoli.
There's a reason our mothers all wanted us to eat our broccoli. The natural immune booster contains vitamins A, C and glutathione.

> "The brain is wider than the sky."
> — *Emily Dickenson*

CHAPTER 8. Engage the brain

Wellness Wake-up Call

You get up every morning at 6:15, take a shower, grab some coffee and a bagel and head off to work, driving the same five miles day in and day out. During the commute, your mind focuses on all the tasks at hand once you get into the office. Your body seems to intuitively know the route. When you pull into the company parking lot, you realize that you don't recall specifics from the last several minutes behind the wheel. You were driving on autopilot.

If you find yourself taking the exact same route to work every day, that's a Wellness Wake-up Call.

8.2

This is your brain...

A popular television ad in the 1980s by a Partnership for a Drug-Free America compared the human brain to an egg.

"This is your brain," the spokesman said, holding up the egg. Then, picking up a frying pan, he added, "This is drugs." After cracking the egg and frying it in the pan, he states, "This is your brain on drugs. Any questions?"

The effective public service announcement definitely got the point across about the dangerous effects drugs can have on the brain, but many everyday things people do — and the things they don't do — can have just as devastating consequences.

Similar commercials could be made for everything from fast food to television to lethargy. Just like our muscles and heart need exercise, nutrition and maintenance, so does the brain.

As the core of the central nervous system, the brain serves like our body's hard drive. Poor lifestyle choices can act like a virus, attacking the brain's functioning until it crashes — and eventually fries.

> "The chief function of the body
> is to carry around the brain."
> — *Thomas A. Edison*

8.3

Cruise and lose

Like drivers can switch on a car's cruise control to maintain a consistent speed while driving highway miles, the brain has similar ways of slipping into auto mode during mundane moments. A study by Daniel Levinson and Richard Davidson of the University of Wisconsin-Madison and Jonathan Smallwood of the Max Planck Institute for Human Cognitive and Brain Science looks at what the researchers refer to as *working memory*, a function of the brain that allows people to juggle multiple thoughts at the same time.

The brain defaults to this mode while we conduct chores like driving a familiar route or taking a shower. Instead of focusing on the task at hand, the mind begins to think about other things, like goals at work or weekend planning. When not focused, the brain allocates resources to the most pressing problems.

Have you ever sat in bed with a good book and despite your interest found that you can't remember the last page you read?

Don't blame the author. Your brain is the culprit.

When your mind starts wandering to other thoughts, resources get redirected and you can lose track of your goals. "It's almost like your attention was so absorbed in the mind wandering that there wasn't any left over to remember your goal to read," Levinson said in the journal *Psychological Science*.

Although people with high-working memory capacity are prone to straying minds, working memory actually can be controlled and used for positive results, like multitasking.

"If your priority is to keep attention on task, you can use working memory to do that too," Levinson added.

But most humans allow themselves to slip into autopilot a majority of their lives — and the results are neither beneficial nor fulfilling. Harvard psychologists Daniel Gilbert and Matthew Killingsworth, conducting research surveying 2,250 volunteers at random intervals, discovered that the average person's mind actually wanders 46.9 percent of the time. During these periods of "mentally checking out," the people surveyed were not focused on a specific task — or even the world around them. Instead, they were caught up in their own thoughts.

While other animals have to focus on specific action and the outside world for survival, humans have become creatures who spend a large majority of life reflecting on events that happened in the past or might happen in the future — or even things that may never happen at all. In fact, mind wandering, according to Gilbert and Killingsworth, appears to be the brain's default mode of operation.

The researchers tracked their volunteers' behavior through a custom-designed iPhone app that contacted each person at random intervals to ask how happy they were, what they were currently doing and whether they were thinking about their current activity or about something else that was pleasant, neutral or unpleasant. "Mind-wandering appears ubiquitous across all activities," Killingsworth said. "This study shows that our mental lives are pervaded, to a remarkable degree, by the nonpresent."

The respondents noted mentally checking out during most of life's activities around 30 percent of the time. The only thing that really held their interest, according to the research, was sex.

The researchers found that people claimed to be the happiest when they were making love, exercising or having a conversation. Unhappiness seemed to be most common during rest, work and using a home computer. "Mind-wandering is an excellent predictor of people's happiness," Killingsworth said. "In fact, how often our minds leave the present and where they tend to go is a better predictor of our happiness than the activities in which we are engaged."

Looking at time-lag analyses, the researchers suggested that their subjects' mind wandering was generally the cause, not the consequence, of much of their unhappiness.

Living in the moment might actually have practical benefits.

"Seize the day, and put the least
possible trust in tomorrow."
— *Horace*

8.4

Doodle or die

Have you ever thought, "I'm so bored I could die?"

Although it might seem a bit far-fetched, boredom actually can be a killer — at least indirectly.

Researchers at University College in London examined questionnaires completed by more than 7,500 London civil servants ages 35 to 55 between 1985 and 1988 that asked if they ever felt bored at work. In a subsequent study, the researchers tracked down how many of the participants in the 1980s survey had died by 2009. According to the report, people who reported they had been very bored were 2.5 times more likely to die of a heart problem than those who hadn't reported being bored.

The report claims that boredom in itself may not be deadly, but it could be a proxy for other risk factors. Sandi Mann, a senior lecturer at the University of Central Lancashire, said that the study correlates with her research that boredom can be linked to anger suppression, which can raise blood pressure and suppress the body's natural immunity.

"People who are bored also tend to eat and drink more, and they're probably not eating carrots and celery sticks," Mann said. Bored people don't invest in learning, growing and challenging their brains, which can speed up the natural degeneration of the brain. Chronic boredom can have serious consequences.

Allowing your brain to automatically slip into autopilot while doing everyday tasks at work or home can lead to future problems, including Alzheimer's and Parkinson's disease. By challenging your brain, you build and strengthen existing neuron connections. Curiosity encourages the brain to stay young.

Even simple diversions away from monotony can be beneficial.

Do you know what Lyndon Johnson, Ronald Reagan, Ralph Waldo Emerson, Barack Obama and Bill Gates all had in common?

They doodled.

Long the disdain of high school algebra teachers, doodling has gotten a bad rap. Although scribbling nonsensical swirls or cartoons in the borders of a notebook might seem like a distraction, it actually can be a focusing technique.

The assumption used to be that a bored brain was inactive, but scientific research has proven quite the opposite.

In a report on the function of doodling published in *Applied Cognitive Psychology*, Jackie Andrade, a professor of psychology at England's University of Plymouth, argues that scribbling actually can help keep our thoughts on target. When people are bored, the brain actually goes into overdrive, according to Andrade. "If you look at people's brain functions when they're bored, we find that they are using a lot of energy — their brains are very active," Andrade said.

The brain is meant to constantly process information, and it demands constant stimulation.

People have been hardwired this way for thousands of years, dating back to the time when humans faced life or death situations every day. Think about the Neanderthals. Predators were a constant threat. "You wouldn't want the brain to just switch off, because a bear might walk up behind you and attack you. You need to be on the lookout for something happening," Andrade said.

Despite modern technology, our brains still function in a similar way. When we aren't being stimulated, the brain searches and scavenges for something to occupy it. This is when people daydream. The downside of daydreaming is that it expends a great deal of energy.

Doodling, on the other hand, allows the brain to multitask. The activity can provide just enough cognitive stimulation during a perceived boring task to stop the brain from seeking more involved stimulation, like fantasies about winning the lottery or breaking up the marriage of Brad Pitt and Angelina Jolie.

To test her theory, the researcher divided a group into two factions — one was instructed to doodle during the task at hand. Andrade then played a tape of a boring telephone message to the subjects. When the tape finished playing, she quizzed both groups on what they had retained.

The doodlers remembered far more than the other subjects — in fact, about 29 percent more. So doodling doesn't detract from concentration because it prevents daydreams, which are the real brain zapper. The next time you find yourself swimming in a sea of numbers at work or finding your attention waning during a meeting, try picking up a pen and scratching a cartoon in the corner or your notepad.

For the brain, doodling is more than Mickey Mouse.

> "I am enough of an artist to draw
> freely upon my imagination."
> — *Albert Einstein*

8.5 Brainology

When it comes to understanding the human brain, most people's knowledge is a little gray.

Although the brain controls everything from being able to do math equations to walking and breathing, the average person tends to take the organ at the core of the central nervous system for granted.

Ironically, we rarely even think about it. Without the brain, there would be no sight, smell, hearing, taste or touch. The essence of who we are as humans wouldn't exist.

In case you were daydreaming in your high school biology class (perhaps you should have doodled more), here's a basic primer on some things you might not remember — or maybe never really knew — about the brain.

At its most basic level, the brain is made up of two kinds of cells: neurons and glial cells. The neurons, which are the basic building block of the nervous system, send and receive nerve impulses or signals. Glial cells, sometimes referred to as the glue of the nervous system, are like a support team, providing nutrition, maintaining homeostatis, forming myelin and aiding in signal transmission. The glial cells are more abundant, outnumbering neurons by about 50 to one.

The tissue in the brain is gray matter or sunstantia grisea. White matter, called sunstantia alba, is composed of nerve fibers, or axons, coated with myelin. In the spinal cord, the white matter is on the surface and the gray matter is inside. In mammals, this pattern is reversed in the brain. Gray matter translates all the sensory information the body receives into chemical data. The axons in white matter act like a messenger service, carrying information from one grey matter region to another.

But the brain isn't simply gray and white. The structure of the organ is divided into regions, and each seems to have its own functions or specializations.

The lower extension of the brain, which connects to the spinal cord, is referred to as the brainstem. Three structures make up the brainstem: the midbrain, the pons and the medulla oblongata. This part of the brain acts like a gateway, passing messages between the various parts of the body and the cerebral cortex, and it houses simple functions we need to survive.

The midbrain helps control eye movement and works with the pons, which coordinates eye and facial movements, facial sensations, hearing and balance. The medulla oblongata works breathing, blood pressure, heart rhythms and swallowing. Because the brainstem controls key functions, damage to it can cause what doctors refer to as *brain death*. The cerebellum, at the back of the brain, works with fine motor skills, like the finger movements used to play a piano. It also controls balance and posture, controlling the equilibrium and the tone of muscles and the position of limbs. You couldn't perform rapid and repetitive action — like those used in playing video games — without the cerebellum.

Most of the brain's real estate is called the cerebrum, which is divided into two major parts: the right and left hemispheres. The surface of the cerebrum contains billions of neurons and glia, which form the cerebral cortex (or gray matter). Each hemisphere can be divided into pairs of frontal, temporal, parietal and occipital lobes.

The frontal lobes are the largest, and they control motor skills, including voluntary movement, speech, and intellectual and behavioral functions. Occipital lobes, at the back of the brain, help humans receive and process visual information, thus influencing how we see and perceive shapes and colors. The parietal lobes interpret signals from other parts of the brain related to vision, hearing, motor, sensory and memory. The temporal lobes on each side of the brain near the ears have unique functions. The right side is connected to visual memory and helps us recognize people's faces and objects. The left works with verbal memory, especially language. The rear of the temporal lobe controls our understanding of others, especially their emotions and reactions.

The hemispheres are what people mean when they discuss "right brain" and "left brain" functions. Generally, the left hemisphere is responsible for language and speech and is often called the dominant side of the brain. The right side dominates when it comes to interpreting visual information and spatial processing.

The words that best describe the left side of the brain are logical, sequential, rational, analytical, objective, systematic, linear, factual, abstract and digital. The right side could be labeled holistic, synthesizing, subjective, non-verbal, casual, visual, sensory, spatial and emotional.

> "It is good to rub and polish
> the brain against that of others."
> — *Michel de Montaigne*

8.6   Did you hear the one about...?

So are you right brained or left brained?

Right-brained people allegedly are creative, intuitive and artistic. Left-brained people are supposed to be linear and logical thinkers who excel at problem solving.

Popular psychology has adopted the concept of right or left brain personalities. The theory originally was inspired by epilepsy research conducted by Roger W. Sperry, who was awarded the Nobel Prize in 1981.

In the subsequent decades, the topic has become the subject of numerous books and self-help movements.

Although based on some fact, the idea of right-brained or left-brained individuals oversimplifies the complexity of the brain, an organ that still holds many mysteries to scientists.

Current imaging science shows that although the brain's hemispheres have specific functions and people are dominant on one side or the other, both sides of the brain are interdependent. The roles are not quite as concrete as previously thought, and the two hemispheres are complementary to each other.

Another common myth involves the percentage of the brain most of us use. A common saying is that average people only use about 10 percent of their brains. In fact, we all use virtually all of our brains on a daily basis. According to Dr. Barry Gordon, a neurologist at Johns Hopkins School of Medicine, the "10 percent myth" is almost laughable.

Even when we are at rest, our brain is in motion. The brain makes up about 3 percent of a person's total weight, but it uses about 20 percent of the body's energy. "It turns out, though, that we use virtually every part of the brain and that (most of) the brain is active almost all the time," Gordon said.

A more accurate statement might be that scientists only understand about 10 percent of how the brain functions. Even some beliefs that were once thought to be facts about the brain are changing as more research data is collected.

Science textbooks used to teach that each person was born with a finite number of brain cells and damage to any of them would mean that an individual would have to function with a deficit for the rest of life.

But brain damage isn't always permanent. Physicians are learning that the brain can repair itself by generating new cells. In addition, the organ also can adapt and compensate for certain losses. The brain actually remains "plastic" throughout life and can change itself in response to new learning and experiences.

> "To think is to practice brain chemistry."
> — *Deepak Chopra*

8.7 Spare some change

Nobody likes change. Your brain is no exception. Much like it's hard to break bad exercise or diet habits, it can be difficult to adopt healthier brain habits.

The brain is trained to operate under what it considers norms. Straying from these routines, or homoestatis, sends out warning signs to the hypothalamus in the brain's core. The hypothalamus, which controls things like thirst, hunger and body temperature, may interpret the change as a stressful event. The brain will want to resist.

Physicians recommend that people who want to make healthier lifestyle choices adopt a slow and steady pace. The brain likes rules, and it won't go into stress mode if positive behaviors are adopted slowly. By practicing healthier choices over and over again for a longer period of time, they will become the new norm. Your brain eventually will decide the new behavior is the one that needs to be protected and continued.

Repetition is key, according to a UCLA study published in the *American Journal of Geriatric Psychology*. Simple lifestyle changes — including memory exercises, better nutrition, exercise and stress reduction — can improve cognitive function and brain efficiency.

After just 14 days of following healthy lifestyle strategies, participants' brain metabolism decreased in working memory regions. The findings suggest an increased efficiency, meaning the brain isn't working as hard to accomplish tasks.

Although once believed that all the ills of youth were what led to brain degeneration later in life, researchers are now seeing that actions in old age are just as important. Engagement is the most important factor, according to Lars Nyberg, a professor of neuroscience at Umea University in Sweden.

In the journal *Trends in Cognitive Science*, Nyberg writes that although genes can play a role, life choices and other environmental factors are critical in old age. Although elderly people do have more trouble remembering meetings or people's names, the memory losses often happen after the age of 60. On the plus side, older people can continue to accumulate knowledge and use what they know effectively.

"There is quite solid evidence that staying physically and mentally active is a way towards brain maintenance," Nyberg said. "Critically, some older adults show little or no brain changes relative to younger adults, along with intact cognitive performance, which supports the notion of brain maintenance. In other words, maintaining a youthful brain, rather than responding to and compensating for changes, may be the key to successful memory aging."

In a study conducted by Dr. Yaakov Stern, a researcher on the causes of Alzheimer's disease, individuals with the greatest levels of leisure activities were 38 percent less likely to develop Alzheimer symptoms. Stern surmises that intellectually stimulating hobbies or activities help build up cognitive reserve, which can postpone the onset of dementia symptoms.

"I like nonsense. It wakes up the brain cells.
Fantasy is a necessary ingredient in living.
It's a way of looking at life through the
wrong end of a telescope — which is what
I do, and that enables you to laugh
at life's realities."
— *Dr. Seuss*

8.8 To thine own brain be true

Brains are as individual as fingerprints. Finding the right strategy to optimize your own brain health requires some self-analysis.

In the publication *Frames of Mind*, psychologist Howard Garner categorized what he describes as individual strengths to help teachers and students understand the spectrum of intelligence. When classifying gifted children, he described seven types of intelligence. Think about which category best describes you.

• *Verbal intelligence* involves the ability to use words. Do you like reading and writing or enjoy crossword puzzles?

- *Visual intelligence* is the ability to imagine things in your mind. Can you see colorful images in your mind, or do you use charts and visuals to make a point?

- *Physical intelligence* involves using your body proficiently. Are you a hands-on kind of person? Do you like to be physically active?

- *Musical intelligence* is the ability to use and understand music. Do you remember tunes or lyrics easily and quickly pick up rhythms?

- *Mathematical intelligence* applies logic to systems and numbers. Are you good at planning and working with numbers?

- *Introspective intelligence* in an understanding your own inner thoughts. Do you enjoy being alone and reflecting on your thoughts?

- *Interpersonal intelligence* is the ability to understand other people and relate well to them. Do you consider yourself people smart?

- Some educators also describe *naturalistic intelligence*, which is sensitivity to living things (think gardeners), and *existential intelligence*, the ability to tackle deep questions about human existence and the meaning of life.

Another interesting point of self-analysis is to determine your learning style, which has practical applications long after you leave school. Our brains pick up cues to process information, and most people tend to use one of their senses more than the others. Which style best describes your most efficient way to retain information?

- *Visual learners* can sit down with a book and easily remember what they have read.

- *Auditory learners* can sit through a lecture and remember key points without taking notes.

- *Kinesthetic learners* might study for a test by taking notes and recopying information until it sticks in their brains.

In the corporate business world, managers may think about their employees based on their critical-thinking type. Although most people may fit into several categories, they usually have one that is more dominant than the others. How do you solve problems? Do you use:

- *Critical thinking*, which involves objectively analyzing a situation by gathering information from a number of sources and then looking at both the tangible and intangible, as well as implications of different courses of action?

- *Implementation thinking*, the ability to organize ideas and plans so they can be carried out effectively?

- *Conceptual thinking*, which finds connections or patterns between abstract ideas and then puts them together to form a bigger picture?

- *Innovative thinking*, or generating new ideas or different ways of approaching things?

- *Intuitive thinking*, a more emotional and sensory approach to understanding a situation?

Understanding the way your brain functions most efficiently can clue you into the best way you solve problems or handle situations. It also can tell you what to do to challenge yourself and get out of autopilot mode.

Comfort zones turn the brain to mush. If you have verbal intelligence, take over the family bookkeeping and challenge yourself with numbers and figures. A visual learner might want to attend a lecture in the community and make a point of paying close attention to every word. Someone who excels at critical thinking should attempt a craft project — break out the hot glue gun and get creative. Doing the opposite of what you do comfortably stimulates the brain, which in turns strengthens it. A mental workout requires change.

8.9

Rapper's delight

This is your brain. This is your brain on rap.

Much like rock 'n' roll was condemned in the 1950s, rap music is often seen in a negative light by people outside the culture. But rappers might be smarter than you think.

The National Institute of Health has collaborated on a project with Los Angeles-based rappers Daniel Rizik-Baer and Michael Eagle to explore the physiological interactions of the mind during "free" rap, an improvisational form of musical poetry.

Researchers Allen Braun and Siyuan Liu of the National Institute on Deafness and Other Disorders asked 12 rappers to memorize a set of lyrics and then rap the words while inside a magnetic resonance machine. The same rappers were then asked to freestyle lyrics to a music track while in the MRI scanner.

When analyzing the images from both sessions, the researchers were surprised by the difference in brain activity. The improvisations showed less activity in parts of the brain usually involved in planning actions and controlling complex behavior, and they showed greater activity in parts of the brain thought to underlie action.

Freestyle rap may involve bypassing a set of cognitive abilities, often called executive function, that allow us to plan and execute complex tasks.

The research also looked at functional connectivity, which shows whether different parts of the brain correlate with one another. A network connecting areas involved in language, emotion and physical movement — and lacking strong connections to areas involved in executive function — showed up during improvisation.

In other words, spontaneous artistic expression might actually change the way your brain functions. Think of it like rerouting an electrical source.

Rapping — or freestyle jazz or other improvisational activities — might even be good for the brain.

"The brain is like a muscle.
When it is in use, we feel very good.
Understanding is joyous."
— Carl Sagan

8.10 Brain health tips

- Get off the couch. Brain health requires stimulation you can't get vegetating for hours in front of the television.

- Focus on nutrition and avoid junk food. Only drink alcohol in moderation.

- Regularly exercise and switch the routine frequently to avoid physical ruts and mental boredom.

- Think about safety. Avoid head injuries by wearing a helmet when riding a bike.

- Manage stress and depression, which research shows actually can damage the brain.

- Get plenty of rest. During deep sleep, the brain repairs itself and boosts the immune system.

- Get regular physicals, and have a physician check blood pressure, heart rate, cholesterol and blood sugar levels.

- Do not smoke or use narcotics. Research suggests that smoking later in life can promote mental decline. It's never too late to quit.

8.11

Brain boosters

Give your brain a boost from some unexpected sources.

① Eat.
Almonds have been connected to memory, and drinking almond oil and milk on a daily basis can strengthen memory power.

② Drink.
Apple juice increases the production of the essential neurotransmitter acetylchlorine in the brain, which can increase memory power

③ Have fun.
All work and no play makes Jack a dull-witted boy. Stress actually drains brainpower by consuming memory resources. Listen to music, play with your children, start writing a blog or take a leisure class.

④ Fast.
Fasting can cleanse and detoxify the body, especially from the stress on the digestive system caused by heavy food. Fasting for a day can strengthen mental clarity, which will aid memory, concentration, creativity and insight

⑤ Exercise your mind.
Challenge yourself by doing crossword puzzles, volunteering at an art gallery, painting or learning a new language. Look for activities outside your comfort zone.

⑥ Meditate.
Meditation and yoga can relieve stress, which is known to be a memory killer.

⑦ Stop the sugar.
Sugar is a carbohydrate with no nutritional value, and excess sugar actually can cause neurotic symptoms, including claustrophobia and memory loss.

⑧ Eat whole wheat.
The lecithin in whole wheat can ease hardening of the arteries, which affects brain function.

"The purpose of life is to live it,
to taste experience to the utmost,
to reach out eagerly and without fear
for newer and richer experience."
—*Eleanor Roosevelt*

CHAPTER 9. Be happier

Wellness Wake-up Call

The alarm rings and you look at the clock begging for 10 more minutes of sleep. You immediately start thinking of everything you have to do today — from getting the kids dressed for school to calling a list of important clients at work — and you dread the next 12 hours. If day-to-day life seems like more of a series of painful chores than interesting adventures, that's a Wellness Wake-up Call.

9.2

Reality rewind

In the 1993 comedy *Groundhog Day*, Bill Murray plays a man caught in a time loop, forced to relive the same 24 hours over and over again until he improves his life — both by helping himself and others. Although the film is played for comedic intent, in actuality, all humans have more in common with Murray's character than they might think. Although we may not find ourselves caught in a literal loop, our actions and emotions repeat more than we probably realize.

Myelin, the same insulating layer around nerves that is linked to our physical health, also plays a role in our emotional and mental well-being.

Have you ever had a friend who always seems to be drawn to unhealthy relationships? Do you know someone who continually yo-yo diets, dropping considerable weight just to regain it by returning to poor eating habits? How many times do you hear people complain about insignificant setbacks in life rather than celebrating positive accomplishments?

Just as our bodies are hard-wired like a computer to follow cycles, so are our emotions. We seem to repeat the same mistakes despite the negative consequences. Although it may appear that we thrive on pain, the reality is that our physiology is caught in a spiral. Bad habits are hard to break because they have become ingrained in our cells. The more we repeat negativity, the more it becomes part of our identity.

An old saying says, "Fool me once, shame on you. Fool me twice, shame on me." Just because harmful emotions have become a constant through life doesn't mean that they have to be your ultimate destiny. Consciously choosing to break a cycle of negativity can be an empowering experience. The only thing you have to lose is misery.

9.3 Practice makes perfect

What separates you from a world-class soccer player?

It might be a lot less than you think.

According to a growing field of scientific research, the success of athletes has as much to do with the brain as it does with brawn. Changes in the brain that take place during repetitive practice at a young age, which are imprinted in myelin, may be the key to athletic ability.

In his popular book, *The Talent Code*, author Daniel Coyle chronicles how myelin attributes to some of the world's "talent hot beds," places that consistently produce winning performers — whether they be on a field or in a symphony. According to Coyle, "Greatness isn't born. It's grown."

Coyle claims that diverse, "talent hot bed" regions of the world — whether producing Brazilian football players or Korean women golfers — have some things in common. The skill acquisition and success foundations are all based on patterns of targeted, deep practice to build skills, which results in accelerated learning.

In other words, coaches have learned to master myelin.

Following *The Talent Code* principle, struggle is an important part of achieving success. Successful people — including the leaders in sports, music and business — all have common traits. They have found the passion to push through difficult challenges and repeat tasks until they become second nature.

By starting slowly with an emphasis on accuracy and repetition, while gradually increasing the difficulty of a drill, performers can bypass bad habits and build myelin pathways that guarantee success. As the myelin gets thicker, we are able to achieve the skill more quickly and with greater accuracy.

But this doesn't just apply to physical movement. All our thoughts and feelings also are precisely timed electrical signals that travel through a chain of neurons wrapped in myelin. With each repetition, the stronger that response becomes. The more we repeat a thought or feeling, the more automatic it becomes.

Our habits, whether good or bad, become part of who we are on a cellular level. Generosity builds generosity. Fear builds fear.

Myelin can either be our best friend or our worst enemy.

"Decisions are the hinges of destiny."
— *Pythagoras*

9.4

Back to the brain

At our core, humans are animals. Much like lions or antelopes, our brains have a built-in safety mechanism to protect us from harm. Often referred to as a fight or flight response, our self-preservation signals are sent through what medical researchers call the limbic system. Based in the brain, the feeling and reacting center can be controlled with our conscious thoughts, but it also responds on its own, saving us from danger before our thinking brain can respond.

The amygdala, an almond-sized and shaped section of the brain, is one of the key components of the limbic system. Although only about an inch long, the structure is linked to our mental and emotional states and controls how we react to

> ### A little experiment
> Watch your language. When you wake up tomorrow, be conscious of your words. Try to make it until lunch without saying any of the following:
>
> No.
> Can't.
> Won't.
> Shouldn't.
> Couldn't.
>
> Notice a difference. Are you able to keep going? If you're able to avoid saying negative words for three weeks, you're guaranteed to come out the other side of those three weeks with an altered and happier perspective on the world.
>
> Make mental note of when others use these words. How do the words affect you when you hear them? How does your use of negative words affect others?

fear, stress and anxiety.

Although our conscious minds can process information about fearful and stressful situations, the amygdala is our brain's visceral reaction. It's that impulse that tells you to get out of the way of a speeding car when you are crossing the street or that instinct that makes you jump when someone accidentally startles you. The amygdala reacts to stimuli and triggers a physiological response that can best be described as the emotion of fear.

In the English language, we often use the terms emotions and feelings interchangeably. But biologically speaking, there is a difference. Feelings are products of the conscious mind. They are labels we give to our unconscious emotions. Emotions are actually distinct patterns of neuron behavior, and they can exist with or without conscious thought.

Fear is the most instinctual and basic emotion. It actually gets imprinted in the amygdala, making frightful experiences specific memories. That's why rethinking a scary event, like a car accident, actually can cause a physiological response. The stressful memory might elicit an increased heart and respiration rate and sweating. Your amygdala is forcing your body to relive the trauma as a defense mechanism.

Although fear, the basest of emotions, is ingrained in our psyche, it's not the only emotion that can become part of our automatic response to outside stimuli. If we frequently face the world with anger or sadness, those emotions will be our initial response to unfamiliar situations.

Similarly, people who have a happier view of life tend to approach each day with optimism.

Do the thing you fear and the death of fear is certain.
— *Ralph Waldo Emerson*

9.5

A myelin carol

It's easier to be Ebenezer Scrooge than Tiny Tim. Our brains are wired that way.

In Charles Dickens' classic, *A Christmas Carol,* the character of Scrooge at first seems like an unsympathetic miser. But as the novella unfolds, we discover his sour disposition actually is the result of years of disappointment and heartache.

Blame myelination for the "Bah! Humbug!"

As Scrooge learns in the morality tale, correcting years of negativity requires conscious change. Although we all want to believe the world is full of good cheer, the word "no" has surprising power. The brain actually has a negative bias, which gives humans a greater sensitivity to unpleasant news. Have you ever wondered why there are so many negative political advertisements during campaign season? It's more than just a case of dirty politics. Psychological research has shown that political smear campaigns are more likely to register in the brain. Similarly, negative news stories have a greater influence than positive ones.

While doing research at Ohio State University, Dr. John Cacioppo showed volunteers three sets of images. One set featured photographs of objects meant to elicit a positive response — this included pictures of sports cars and pizza. Another grouping focused on the negative, including dead animals. A third showed more neutral images, like a dinner plate and a hair dryer.

Cacioppo recorded electrical activity in the cerebral cortex during the experiment. According to the results, the research subjects' brains reactivated most strongly to stimuli perceived of as negative — with a greater surge in electrical activity.

In fact, just seeing the word *no* for less than one second can release dozens of stress-producing hormones and neurotransmitters. The chemicals immediately interrupt the normal functions of the brain — logic, reason, language processing and communication are disrupted.

Add a frown, and the word has even stronger impact. More stress chemicals are released in the brain of the speaker, and anyone listening also will experience an increase in anxiety and irritability. Negativity can poison both your own mind and the thoughts of people around you.

Through myelination, negativity becomes a habit. The more you engage in negative conversations, the harder it is to have positive thoughts and feelings. And when you allow anger to rule your thoughts and actions, the decision-making centers in the frontal lobe of your brain get out of whack. The angrier you get, the more likely you are to act irrationally.

Some of this propensity toward the negative probably goes back to cave man days. Thousands of years ago, this negativity kept us safe. Before modern civilization, the species' survival depended on dodging danger. The brain naturally developed in a way that would make it unavoidable not to notice danger — and to force us to get out of harm's way.

But barring a resurgence in the population of wooly mammoths, humans no longer need the negative myelin threads that have become part of our DNA. It's time to put down the clubs.

> There is little difference in people,
> but that little difference makes a big difference.
> The little difference is attitude.
> The big difference is whether it is positive or negative.
> — *W. Clement Stone*

9.6 Happy genes

Could our disposition in life really be the result of generations of emotions? Scientific research is discovering that our parents — and our parents' parents — play an enormous role in whether we are happy or sad. In fact, close to one-half of our sense of well-being is inherited. Scientists at UCLA have linked the oxytocin receptor gene to optimism and self-esteem. People missing certain nucleotides in the gene are more likely to have a pessimistic attitude.

Another study by psychologists at the University of Edinburgh and the Queensland Institute for Medical Research in Australia backs up the data by using a personality test called the Five-Factor Model. Administered to nearly

1,000 pairs of twins, the test measured the subjects' happiness and amount of time spent worrying and found evidence for common genes that predispose people to happiness.

"Although happiness is subject to a wide range of external influences, we have found that there is a heritable component of happiness which can be entirely explained by genetic architecture of personality," said Alexander Weiss of the University of Edinburgh, one of the leaders of the study.

David Lykken, a professor emeritus at the University of Minnesota, found correlating figures in another twin study. According to Lykken's research, when twins were separated at birth, 60 percent of them described themselves as happy, despite environmental differences.

Several twin studies also have linked depression to heredity by about 40 percent. Does that mean that we are predestined to be either happy or sad? Not exactly. Although the research links emotions to heredity, none of the studies take our conscious choices and environmental factors out of the equation.

Scientists in the UCLA study, for example, emphasize that the effects of the "happy gene" are far from an absolute. Although babies born with the gene for green eyes will have green eyes, the same is not true when it comes to happiness. Everything from nurturing, love, friendships, therapy and physical activity can influence oxytocin levels. When it comes to depression, biology isn't necessarily destiny. Every child born has about a 16.5 percent chance to experience a depressive episode at some point in life.

Our heredity only predisposes us to happiness or depression. About 50 percent in the differences between people's emotional states can be linked to external factors, including relationships, health and careers. Genetics is not black-and-white when it comes to emotions, and individuals have the power to rewire their genes.

"These then are my last words to you.
Be not afraid of life.
Believe that life is worth living
and your belief will help create the fact."
— *William James*

9.7

Turn that frown upside down

A Bing Crosby hit from 1944, written by Harold Arlen and Johnny Mercer, encouraged people to *Ac-Cent-Tchu-Ate the Positive*. According to the song's lyrics, "You've got to accentuate the positive. Eliminate the negative. Latch on to the affirmative. Don't mess with Mister In-Between." The swing-era ditty may be a catchy tune, but its affirmative mantra actually has some scientific backbone. You just might have to sing it three times to really benefit.

Because our brains have a natural negative bias, positive thoughts don't come easily. Positive messages are not a threat to our survival (think back to that caveman ancestor), so our brains don't feel an immediate need to respond. In fact, positive thoughts require conscious and repetitive attempts to break through. Barbra Frederickson, one of the founders of the Positive Psychology movement, actually found scientific evidence that people need to generate at least three positive thoughts or feelings to overcome one expression of negativity.

Put the theory to the test. Think about the last time you looked in the mirror. Which thought had the most weight? "I'm having a good hair day today," or "I look fat." Some people might be surprised to learn just how important words can be. According to Frederickson, repeating positive words like love, peace and compassion will turn on specific genes that can help lower physical and emotional stress.

Having a positive influence on others can be even more difficult. The research indicates that effective personal and business relationships require at least five positive messages for each negative expression — including body language like frowns and nods of the head. So unfortunately, the word *yes* has only about 20 percent of the power of *no*.

> "The life I touch for good or ill
> will touch another life,
> until who knows where the
> trembling stops or in what far
> place my touch will be felt."
> —*Frederick Beuchner*

9.8

Til negativity do us part

Want to know the key to a happy marriage? It has little to do with perfectly chiseled features, chemistry or even occasional weekend getaways. It's a numbers game.

Around half of all American marriages end in divorce, and it has more to do with attitude than any major crisis, like the breaking of vows or a financial meltdown. Several scientific studies have found that the marriages with the greatest longevity manage to focus on the positive.

That's not to say that people who stay together live in constant bliss, but the good times do outweigh the bad — by around five to one. Even couples who bicker and seem to frequently argue can stay together if they meet the magic quota.

Scientific data suggests that as long as spouses have five times as many more positive feelings and interactions than negative, the marriage will be stable. According to the research, couples who divorce have spent more time on the negative. Even a relationship that is 50 to 60 percent positive is destined to fail.

And the odds can't be swung in the other direction by grand gestures. A large event, like a birthday or anniversary party, might be nice, but it won't salvage an unhealthy relationship. However, a loop of little things — like a kind word or a greeting card — might do the trick. Consistent appreciation and positive recognition has a profoundly positive effect on a relationship. Researchers have found that frequent, small acts matter most.

"Positive anything is better than negative nothing."
— *Elbert Hubbard*

9.9
Optimism has its advantages

Finding the glass half full instead of empty will do more than help you win a congeniality award. It actually can be the difference between success and failure.

According to researcher Suzanne Segerstrom, a specialist in positive psychology, attitude has as much to do with our accomplishments as skill and hard work. Although we all encounter failures and disappointments in life, optimists are more likely to work through their problems and push ahead.

"Setbacks are inherent to almost every worthwhile human activity, and a number of studies show that optimists are in general both psychologically and physiologically healthier," Segerstrom said.

When faced with stress, optimists are better at coping than pessimists. When faced with a disappointment, optimists are more likely to objectively look at the situation and search for a solution. Pessimists are more likely to feel out of control and just give up. Research shows that optimists are more likely to be successful at the jobs. Their positive attitudes help them gain empowerment, and their personal initiative opens up more opportunities.

"We found that optimism is the greatest predictor of entrepreneurial success because it allows your brain to perceive more possibilities," said Shawn Achor, author of the book *The Happiness Advantage* "Only 25 percent of job success is based upon IQ. Seventy-five percent is about how your brain believes your behavior matters, connects to other people and manages stress."

The same principles apply to personal relationships. Optimists also tend to be happier in their marriages, possibly because they bring more positivity than negativity to their partners. In addition, they are more likely to raise resilient kids, who will be able to make healthy choices without helicopter parenting.

The benefits of optimism are more than half-full — they are overflowing. Overall, optimists tend to be healthier. Looking at the effects of negativity on the effectiveness of flu vaccines, researchers found that negative emotions lead to a weaker response. Optimists, on the other hand, saw a greater immune response. According to the Mayo Clinic, optimism also is associated with a longer lifespan and a reduced risk of depression and cardiovascular disease.

In a study by the Harvard School of Public Health, researcher Julia Boehm found that optimistic people have half the risk of having a first heart attack. Optimists in the research group also had healthier blood pressure, cholesterol and weight. The research indicated that the stress associated with negative psychological traits could lead to damage of both the arteries and the heart.

And the benefits of your positive disposition extend beyond yourself — and even your immediate family. Happiness is a like a virus, and it is much easier to spread than the common cold. If one person in a group expresses happiness, researchers have been able to measure a three-degree spread of that emotion — even reaching out to absolute strangers.

"Especially in the United States, we're very used to thinking of ourselves as rugged individuals. But even very small things that happen to us have big impacts on dozens and hundreds of other people," said James Fowler, a University of California, San Diego political scientist who co-authored a study with Harvard University medical sociologist Nicholas Christakis. The study examined nearly 5,000 people over the course of 20 years. For an average person, every person in a social network increases the chance of personal happiness by 9 percent, and the contagious effects of happiness last up to one year.

According to the research, when someone gets happy, that person's friends experience a 25 percent increased chance of improved emotions. A friend of that friend will have a nearly 10 percent chance of added happiness — and a friend of that friend has a 5.6 percent chance in the gain of positive feelings.

Even a stranger's good mood can do more for your happiness than receiving a $5,000 raise, which, according to the researchers, only increases happiness by about 2 percent.

> "We must look for the opportunity in every difficulty instead of being paralyzed by the difficulty in every opportunity."
> — *Walter E. Cole*

9.10

Second that emotion

Don't blame drugs. Blame the endorphins.

Although addicts become hooked on substances like morphine and cocaine, in reality, they are really craving the feeling they get from endorphins, neurotransmitters that interact with the opiate receptors in the brain to reduce the perception of pain. Secretions of endorphins can provide a feeling of euphoria. They are responsible for the "runner's high" people get while exercising.

In addition to strenuous physical activity, endorphins are released during sex, while meditating and even from eating certain foods, including spicy peppers and chocolate. Recent research shows that laughter can send the same feel-good impulses to the brain.

"We think it is the bonding effects of the endorphin rush that explain why laughter plays such an important role in our social lives," said Robin Dunbar, a researcher from the University of Oxford.

According to Dunbar's study, people are able to tolerate more pain after laughing, especially if they had laughed with a group of other people. Watching about 15 minutes of comedy with other people increased the subjects' pain thresholds by 10 percent. The results were slightly smaller for people who had watched comedies alone.

Another laughter study, which monitored the brain activity of people reading comic strips, found that humorous punch lines actually activated a network of regions of the

Changes In Attitude

Want to adopt a more optimistic attitude? You can't switch from being a pessimist to an optimist overnight, but you can make the change in less than a month. Try this simple exercise.

Each morning when you get up, write down three things in your life that make you grateful. Repeat this exercise for three weeks.

"What we found was that something as simple as writing down three things that you are grateful for every day for 21 days in a row significantly increases your level of optimism and it holds for the next six months," Achor found while researching *The Happiness Advantage*.

brain, including the amygdala. Extremely funny clips resulted in more blood flow to the area, thus stimulating the reward center.

"The finding is potentially significant in terms of understanding normal variation in personality and behavior as well as certain brain disorders, such as depression," said Dr. Allan Reiss, director of the Stanford Psychiatry Neuroimaging Laboratory and co-director of the Center for Brain and Behavior at Packard Children's Hospital.

The study indicated that the same part of the brain that can be negatively influenced through drug addiction could evolve to enhance learning and behavior through positive feedback, such as laughter. Although happiness and laughter certainly have their rewards, people shouldn't expect eternal bliss. Feelings of sadness or stress can be important signals. Moments of unhappiness or mild depression might actually serve a social purpose.

"Let's say you're moving through positions of increasing responsibility at work," said neurobiologist Robin Lester. "You might get to a point where it's too much. That level is different for each person, so depression —lowering your level of happiness — might be your brain's way of indicating that you're not at the level that's best for you."

If laughter is good for the brain, does that mean that crying is detrimental? Not necessarily. Although long-term sadness usually is an indication of depression, occasional tears are part of normal life — and may even have their own benefits.

Most healthy people report a feeling of catharsis after a cry. The tears have a purifying emotional release. In fact, an international sample of men and women from 30 different countries found that most reported feeling relief after a good cry. Another study, reviewing more than 3,000 reports of recent crying episodes, noted that the majority of the subjects even reported an improvement in their mood afterward. However, people with mood disorders, clinical depression or anxiety problems are less likely to feel better after crying.

Some conditions are more conducive to crying than others. For example, people who receive social support while crying tend to feel better about the experience than people who cry alone. But crying in public isn't recommended. Make sure you feel comfortable and are in a location where you won't experience shame or embarrassment. Also, crying after a problem is solved is more effective than shedding tears before you have dealt with a situation, which can lead to even more negative emotions.

Perpetual optimism is a force multiplier.
— *Colin Powell*

9.11   Meditate on this

Being thick-headed can have positive benefits.

Neuroscientists have discovered that people who practice regular meditation have measurably thicker brains in key regions, including the insula and the prefrontal cortex. The areas are centers for deep feelings and focusing and attention. In addition, meditation slows the loss of brain cells through cortical thinning. The average person has lost about 4 percent of total brain mass by the time he or she reaches 80. For people who meditate, that figure is considerably lower.

Meditation can physically change the brain.

A Massachusetts General Hospital study of the brain scans of 16 people found that the positive effects of meditation could be surprisingly rapid. After just an eight-week course of mindfulness meditation, the subjects' brains showed obvious changes. The parts of the participants' brains associated with compassion and self-awareness grew, and the sections affiliated with stress actually shrank.

Researchers at the University of Wisconsin found more interesting data after looking at the brains of long-time meditators — the Dalai Lama's monks. Using high-tech equipment, the scientists scanned the monks' brains during meditation. The subjects' electroencephalogram patterns, which measure the electrical activity in the brain, increased and remained higher during the process. Despite the restful state, the brain was more active.

The positive effects of meditation last beyond the process itself. When a professor at Emory University recorded conversations of people who regularly practiced meditation, they found surprisingly positive results.

"They were more empathetic with people," said Chuck Raison, who conducted the study. "They were spending more time with other people. They laugh more, you know, all those things. They didn't use the 'I' as much. They use the word 'we' more."

9.12   Not a yogi yet...but you must start somewhere

You may be experienced at meditating or a novice. If you'd like to learn more, abundant resources exist, but here are some basic tips for meditating.

(1) Sit on the ground, if possible — lotus position not required. If you don't sit on the ground/floor, sit in a chair with both feet on the floor.

(2) Think about the vertebrae in your spine. Starting with the bottom of your spine, start stacking each on the one below it. This will have you sitting perfectly balanced and you should find it easy to maintain and relaxing. For starters, let your arms just hang.

(3) Close your eyes and try to relax your whole body. Do a mental scan of your body to find parts that may not be completely relaxed. When identified, relax that part.

(4) Focus only on breathing in and out. The big idea of meditating is to silence your mind. If (and when) things float into your mind, don't chastise yourself. Just let the thoughts go and focus on your breathing. Some people like to count their breaths.

(5) Start with five minutes. Work up to 30.

"No man is an island."
—John Donne

CHAPTER 10.   Relationships

Wellness Wake-up Call

List the people in your inner circle. How many did you name? Now define your inner circle. Are they people you trust with your deepest and darkest moments? Would you trust them with your children? Do you find yourself endlessly scrolling through Facebook feeling like life is passing you by? You might "like" a cute kitten photo or make a brief comment on a high school chum's recent vacation shots, but most of your online time is spent feeling isolated rather than loved.

Despite having hundreds of online "friends," day-to-day life seems impersonal and lonely.

Do you feel alone much of the time? If loneliness has become a daily emotion for you, that's a Wellness Wake-up Call.

10.2

A little less face time

Thirty years ago, if you wanted to get in touch with a friend or loved one, you had to go visit them face to face, pick up the telephone and make a phone call or even write a letter or postcard.

Today, communication has become more immediate and streamlined. We can reach the entire world in a matter of seconds.

We use smart phones — kept within reach every minute of the day — to Tweet brief thoughts. We post philosophical observations and vent rants online through Facebook, where we are connected to hundreds, maybe thousands of people through a network of "friends."

We continually send out messages, but how often do we truly communicate?

Telephone calls are becoming a rarity for younger generations, who prefer to text message by cell phone with emoticons rather than real words.

Even when we give each other face time, we rarely disconnect from technology. Couples sit at restaurant tables checking status updates rather than talking about their days. Family time is more about iPads than conversation.

The more we plug into the world, the less connected we truly are.

"On Twitter, we get excited when someone follows us. In real life, we get scared and run away."
— *unknown*

10.3

The trouble with 'friends'

In 2011, Facebook tracked 845 million users — that's a lot of *friends*. In the last three months of that year, the social media site's users posted 2.7 billion comments and *likes* every day. One out of every 13 people in the world has at least one Facebook account — and more than half of the website's users log on daily. For people ages 18 to 34, the statistics are even more staggering. Nearly half the people in that age group check Facebook minutes after waking up and 28 percent admit to logging on before they even get out of bed.

But despite this technological connection, researchers are finding that people feel less linked to their fellow humans. Even before the launch of social media, scientists were noting a change. In 1998, a research team at Carnegie Mellon University documented that increased Internet usage (and this was back in the day of dial-up) coincided with a rise in perceived loneliness. Sociologists have dubbed the phenomenon the Internet paradox.

Although humans have more opportunity and tools to communicate than in any other time in the history of the world, the average person has few significant relationships. In the past, most people lived in family units, but household sizes have continually declined in the last 60 years. In 1950, less than 10 percent of all homes were single-person households. Today, nearly 27 percent of all households are single-person. Living alone has become a norm.

In 1985, the average person had 2.94 people he or she considered to be personal confidants. Less than 20 years later, that number had dropped to 2.08. Around 10 percent of Americans in 1985 said they had nobody they felt comfortable enough with to share important details, and 15 percent claimed to only have one close friend. Two decades later, 25 percent of people surveyed admitted that they had no one they considered a confidant, and 20 percent said they only had one close friend.

As more people live alone, the chance for human interaction decreases. Single people may have daily discussions with co-workers and spend an occasional evening out with a friend, but once they come home at night, they are isolated. Many people turn to Facebook and other social media sites for contact with the outside world, but Internet socializing has limitations and consequences.

Researchers in Australia, a country where half the population uses Facebook, found that people who described themselves as lonely tended to spend more time on the social networking site. But which came first, the loneliness or the Facebook use? Although the report couldn't document that the site causes loneliness, they definitely saw some interesting correlations.

For the study, the researchers described social loneliness as a sense of not feeling bonded with friends. In the people surveyed, Facebook users actually had slightly lower levels of social loneliness than people who didn't use the social media site. However, Facebook users had significantly higher levels of family loneliness, the sense of not feeling connected to family members.

Moira Burke, a researcher at the Human-Computer Institute at Carnegie Mellon, found that the way people use Facebook also has some effect on their emotions. People who passively scan the site, looking at friends' status updates and making posts on their own walls — tended to feel more disconnected. Hitting the like button and commenting on friends' posts brings users more satisfaction, according to the study. Personalized messages brought the greatest satisfaction.

"People who received compound communication became less lonely, while people who received one-click communication experienced no change in loneliness," Burke said. "People whose friends write to them semi-publicly on Facebook experience decreases in loneliness."

Sherry Turkle, a professor of computer culture at MIT, writes about the phenomenon in her book, *Alone Together*.

"These days, insecure in our relationships and anxious about intimacy, we look to technology for ways to be in relationships and protect ourselves from them at the same time. The ties we form through the Internet are not, in the end, the ties that bind. But they are the ties that preoccupy. We don't want to intrude on each other, so instead we constantly intrude on each other, but not in 'real time,'" Turkle writes.

The main point is that building a long list of *friends* on Facebook won't bring happiness in the non-virtual world. John Cacioppo, director of the Center for Cognitive and Social Neurosciences at the University of Chicago and the author of the book *Loneliness*, emphasizes that people shouldn't confuse digital *friends* with true relationships. People with strong networks of friends will transfer that depth to their circle of friends on the online social network. People who are lonely when they are not logged on are just as likely to feel disconnected on Facebook — no matter how many *likes* they experience on a daily basis.

*"The most terrible poverty is loneliness,
and the feeling of being unloved."*
—Mother Teresa

10.4   Only the lonely

One isn't necessarily the loneliest number.

Married people can be lonely. Children who live in a house with five siblings can fell loneliness. Celebrities, adored by millions of eager fans, might even feel that they are all alone deep inside — yet someone who lives alone might not describe himself as lonely.

Loneliness is a psychological, rather than a physical, state of being.

About 60 million people, or about 20 percent of Americans, are unhappy because of loneliness. Living in a culture that emphasizes the importance of happiness hasn't made people any happier. In fact, according to one study, it may have the reverse outcome.

Researchers at the University of Denver found a paradox in our desire for happiness. Under conditions of low life stress, people who want to be happy are less likely to find satisfaction. In fact, according to the report, they will have lower psychological well-being and life satisfaction. They also will be more likely to have symptoms of depression.

But can loneliness be measured? Scientists at UCLA have created a tool to define the condition. Dubbed the UCLA Loneliness Scale, the test asks a series of 20 questions that all begin with "How often do you feel ...?" How do you think you would measure?

UCLA Loneliness Scale Instructions:

Mark the letter following each question that best describes your emotions. Use the following key:

O = I often feel this way.
S = I sometimes feel this way.
R = I rarely feel this way.
N = I never feel this way.

	O	S	R	N
How often do you feel unhappy doing so many things alone?				
How often do you feel you have nobody to talk to?				
How often do you feel you cannot tolerate being so alone?				
How often do you feel as if nobody really understands you?				
How often do you find yourself waiting for people to call or write?				
How often do you feel completely alone?				
How often do you feel you are unable to reach out and communicate with those around you?				
How often do you feel starved for company?				
How often do you feel it is difficult for you to make friends?				
How often do you feel shut out and excluded by others?				
YOUR TOTAL				
	x4	x3	x2	x1
ADD TOTALS FOR LONELINESS SCORE				

Instructions: Scores between 15 and 20 are considered a normal experience of loneliness. Scores above 30 indicate a person is experiencing severe loneliness.

10.5   Loneliness is bad for your health

Loneliness can lead to depression and suicide, cardiovascular disease and stroke, increased stress levels, decreased memory and learning ability, antisocial behavior, poor decision-making, alcoholism and drug abuse, the progression of Alzheimer's disease and altered brain function.

Since loneliness is a psychological state, it starts in our brain. Although social interactions are emotional rather than physical, they do have physiological effects on our bodies. The simple act of cooperation activates the reward section of the brain in the same way as hunger is satiated with food. Social rejection actually registers in the brain as pain, according to neurologists, and even empathy can be read in magnetic resonance images.

The feeling of loneliness actually is a message from our brain motivating us to reconnect with other humans. If we ignore these signals, they can become ingrained in our DNA and lead to depression and poor physical health.

According to Cacioppo, people who described themselves as lonely actually show physical implications in testing.

"When we drew blood from our older adults and analyzed their white cells, we found that loneliness somehow penetrated the deepest recesses of the cell to alter the way the genes were being expressed," he writes.

Extreme loneliness even can be passed on to future generations. A Dutch study of twins showed that loneliness could be as genetically linked as neuroticism and anxiety.

> "The trouble is not that I am single and likely to stay single,
> but that I am lonely and likely to stay lonely."
> —*Charlotte Brontë*

10.6

Fortress of Solitude

Solitaire is meant to be played alone, but that doesn't mean that people who master the card game are inherently lonely.

There is a big difference between loneliness and solitude.

Have you ever walked though a shopping mall surrounded by hundreds of strangers yet felt utterly isolated? On the flip side, have you ever been snuggled up in bed by yourself reading a mystery novel and felt like the center of the universe?

There can be comfort in being alone, but much of it has to do with self-acceptance. While loneliness is a negative state, solitude is a positive and constructive frame of mind. When people experience solitude, alone time is a cherished escape from the noise of the world.

Solitude is a chance for the body and mind to reconnect without distractions from other people. While loneliness may seem like a punishment, solitude should feel like a reward. Solitude is alone time that promotes self worth, which is a necessary component of true intimacy in relationships.

Ways to achieve solitude:

- Turn off the television, computer and other electronic devices.
- Relax and read a book without interruption.
- Find a new recipe and prepare it in leisure without the stress of having to cook a family meal.
- Meditate.
- Take a walk by yourself, especially in an area surrounded by nature.
- Soak in the bathtub.
- Complete an art or craft project.
- Garden.
- Exercise.

10.7

Can you relate?

Think of all the words other people in your life could use to identify you: best friend, mother, neighbor, co-worker, daughter, sister, wife, client, and classmate. Relationships refer to the way we *connect* with each other. We have a relationship with every person we meet, whether it is superficial or evolves into something much deeper. Although other animals form social relationships, none are as complex as what human culture has developed through thousands of years of history.

Although some relationships are chosen, others are thrust upon us. For example, a friend is someone that we consciously choose to be around because they bring us happiness and fulfillment. Family, on the other hand, has a more structured purpose. Family members help us establish roles and identities and shape our growth. Romantic relationships bring us passion, intimacy and commitment. Professional relationships are about cooperation and attaining similar goals in a structured setting. Your body language may tell you more than you might imagine about your relationships. An episode of the classic sitcom *Seinfeld* once coined the term "close-talker" for a person who invaded interpersonal space by getting too close during conversations. Although personal space might seem like an abstract concept, scientists actually have delineated four zones people commonly use in relationships.

When we are intimately involved with someone, we are comfortable having them within 18 inches or less of our personal space. That space extends farther out depending on the type of relationship. Personal relationships, like friends, are best kept at about 1 ½ to 4 feet. People we are social with, like co-workers, should stay about 4 to 12 feet from us. Strangers make us uncomfortable when they get closer than 12 feet. Of course, these numbers are generalized. Every person has his or her own personal bubble, and the amount of space could be different from friend to friend. The relationships we foster — whether they be friendly, familial, romantic or professional — provide support. Healthy relationships involve people we feel comfortable being around whom we feel like we can tell anything. A good relationship gives you a source for problem solving and makes you feel valued and that your concerns are being taken seriously. People in positive relationships offer each other concrete help, emotional support, a different perspective, advice and validation.

Relationships, however, do require work.

10.8

Tips for a healthy relationship

No one will ever be exactly what you want — in any kind of relationship. Make sure you always keep your expectations realistic. Everyone is bound to disappoint us at one point or another. Communication is key. Take the time to really talk — and genuinely listen to what the other person has to say. Sharing is central to building and fostering trust. Relationships change over time, and people need to remain flexible so they can grow and prosper.

Don't be a martyr. Treating yourself well is an important part of maintaining healthy relationships. Be reliable. When you make plans, stick to them. Conflicts will arise, but remember to fight fair. If things get heated, negotiate another time to talk when you both can relax and reflect. When you do have a conversation, don't criticize. Address the issue rather than attacking the person, and don't place blame. If both parties can't see eye-to-eye, sometimes it's best to agree to disagree and call a truce. Most importantly, don't hold a grudge. Be emotionally present and show warmth. Maintain a balance in your life so you will have time to foster relationships. Don't try to be what you think someone else wants. Be yourself. Relationships won't fulfill you unless you feel like you are valued for whom you really are.

> "may came home with a smooth round stone
> as small as a world and as large as alone."
> —*e.e. cummings*

10.9

The friend zone

Although the number of confidants the average person has in his or her life has shrunk in the last century, that doesn't mean we are all destined to loneliness. Friendship is more about quality than quantity. According to psychologists, a few friendships that are close and meaningful have greater benefit than a mass of superficial social connections.

According to Rebecca G. Adams, a professor of sociology at the University of North Carolina at Greensboro, friendships are the most important relationships people have.

"In general, the role of friendship in our lives isn't terribly well appreciated," Adams said. "Friendship has a bigger impact on our psychological well-being than family relationships."

When it comes to friends, is there a magic equation? Possibly, according to anthropologist Robin Dunbar. The researcher developed an assessment, often referred to as Dunbar's number, to define the number of relationships humans are cognitively capable of maintaining. Dunbar's number is 150.

That figure, however, is based on real-time friends. In the social media world, different rules apply. According to Facebook, the average friend count is 190. The site's in-house sociologist, Cameron Marlow, suggests that 302 is the ideal number. Marlow points out that a woman with 500 Facebook friends only interacts regularly with a fraction of that number — she might post comments on the pages of about 26 and truly communicate with around 16. A man with 500 friends is likely to post comments on 17 pages and communicate with 10. So even if you build a network of *friends* in the online world, that doesn't mean that your social activity is increasing. Facebook's own research indicates that quantity doesn't correlate with quality. Real-time friends may be able to offer a shoulder to cry on, but their benefits go far deeper than emotional support. In fact, a number of scientific studies document that having strong friendships can improve your health and increase your chances of living to an older age. Friendships can help you fight illness and depression, speed up recovery times and slow the aging process.

In 2006, researchers followed nearly 3,000 nurses who had breast cancer to see if relationships had any affect on their recovery. The study found that women without any close friends were four times as likely to die from the disease than women who said they had 10 or more friends.

Similarly, David Spiegel, a professor of psychology at Stanford University, documented that women with breast cancer who participated in support groups lived twice as long as those who didn't go to meetings — and they also said they had considerably less pain.

An Australian research team at the Centre for Ageing Studies at Flinders

University followed nearly 1,500 older people for 10 years to see how social interactions correlated with health. The results showed that the subjects who had a large network of friends outlived those with fewer friends by 22 percent.

According to Life Extensions, a nonprofit dedicated to research on extending the human life span, social isolation can be just as negative as the worst personal habits. For example, not having friends is as bad for your health as smoking 15 cigarettes a day, as dangerous as being an alcoholic, as harmful as never exercising and twice as dangerous as obesity.

"Friends help you face adverse events. They provide material aid, emotional support and information that helps you deal with the stressors," said Sheldon Cohen, a psychology professor at Carnegie Mellon University. "There may be broader effects as well. Friends encourage you to take better care of yourself. And people with wider social networks are higher in self-esteem, and they feel they have more control over their lives."

Increase your sense of belonging and purpose

- Boost your happiness
- Reduce stress
- Improve your self-worth
- Help you cope with traumas, such as divorce, serious illness, job loss or the death of a loved one
- Encourage you to change or avoid unhealthy lifestyle habits, including excessive drinking or physical inactivity

10.10 One is silver and the other is gold

Making friends seems to get harder as we grow older, but perhaps adults could learn a few lessons from children. A team of researchers at the University of California at Riverside found that pre-teens who performed deliberate acts of kindness were more popular with their peers. In the study, the researchers assigned three acts of kindness to the children each week for four weeks, and the kind deeds were not necessarily directed toward their classmates. Examples included giving Mom a hug when she feels stressed about her job, giving someone some of my lunch and vacuuming the floor.

The team worked with 400 children between the ages of 9 and 11. Before the acts of kindness began, the researchers had each student circle the names of students from their classroom that they would like to join in school activities. Four weeks later, the children were asked to repeat the nomination process. Students who had practiced acts of kindness gained significantly more nominations. Kinder children were more popular.

"The most interesting finding to me is that a simple positive activity can promote positive relationships among peers," said Kristin Layous, a researcher with the project.

"The family.
We were a strange little band
of characters trudging through life
sharing diseases and toothpaste,
coveting one another's desserts,
hiding shampoo, borrowing money,
locking each other out of our rooms,
inflicting pain and kissing to heal it in the
same instant, loving, laughing, defending,
and trying to figure out the common thread
that bound us all together."
— *Erma Bombeck*

10.11

We are family

As social networks shrink, the importance of family may be on the rise. In a study published in the American Sociological Review, researchers reported that between 1985 and 2004, the number of Americans who talk about serious matters only to family members increased from 57 percent to 80 percent. Family relationships also play an important role in our physical well-being. Living alone is bad for your health. According to the National Center for Health Statistics at the Centers for Disease Control and Prevention, married men and women in all age groups are less likely to be limited in activity due to illness. Middle-aged adults living alone have higher rates of doctor visits, acute conditions and both short and long-term disability.

Looking at 225 newlywed couples, researchers at the University of Massachusetts noticed physical indicators of emotional bonds. According to the data, the way people feel attached to each other affects cortisol levels in response to stress. The response could be a predictor of depression and anxiety over time, and the research indicates that the emotional aspects of relationships can influence future mental health challenges.

If you don't think our close relationships have an effect on our physiology, take this study into consideration. Psychologist Robert Zajonc found that people who live with each other for 25 years actually develop similar facial features. It's not that people chose partners who look like them. The research actually documents noticeable changes in appearance over time. In the study, 110 subjects were shown individual photographs of newlyweds. Then they examined pictures of the same people after 25 years of marriage. Both sets of photos were cropped so that only the faces were visible, and the participants did not know the marital status of the people in the images. Surprisingly, the participants matched photos of people who had been married for a quarter century merely by their resemblance to each other.

The researchers have several theories on why people might begin to look alike after years together. Diet is one option. Perhaps sharing a similar diet over time could result in the change, but a smaller study by the scientists showed no significant correlation. The researchers also looked at environmental factors, like the affects of sunshine on the skin. But again, that theory was disproved because all of the subjects were from the exact same region of the country and were exposed to similar climates. A third hypothesis was that people were predisposed to choose partners who will grow to look like them. Perhaps, for example, depressed people are attracted to each other, so over time, both look depressed. But what the authors think to be the most likely cause is empathy. People start to resemble each other because they empathize with their spouse and subconsciously mimic each other's facial expressions. The repetition over time results in the morphing of facial features.

Our spouse's health also can affect our own physical well-being. Joelle Ruthig, a researcher at the Department of Psychology at the University of North Dakota, found that spouses with impaired partners were likely to develop their own health and psychological problems. The study looked at 71 married couples in their 70s and assessed facts over a two-year period. Ruthig found that men were more greatly affected. The husbands with the best health also had wives who were highly functioning.

Husbands with sick wives often suffered both physical and mental setbacks. On the flip side, the health of husbands had less impact on the well-being of wives, especially their mental health. Researchers theorized that perhaps because women traditionally play the role of caregiver in families, having to care for an aging spouse was less stressful.

Even the healthiest relationships experience some rough spots. Arguments can be stressful on a relationship, but they can be just as harmful on the individual's health. A study from the University College London found that individuals who experienced high levels of negativity in personal relationships, especially marriage, were 1.34 times more likely to experience cardiovascular issues, including chest pain, heart attacks and even sudden cardiac death. The study looked at 9,000 British civil servants and noted negative marital interactions and their link to depression and anger. Over time, the negative emotions added a cumulative "wear and tear" effect on vital organs, notably the heart.

"I am fond of pigs.
Dogs look up to us.
Cats look down on us.
Pigs treat us as equals."
— *Winston Churchill*

10.12

Working it out

The average person spends 90,000 hours at work during their lifetime, and 80 percent of people surveyed about job satisfaction said they were dissatisfied with their employment. A study from Chartered Management Institute and Workplace Health Connect reports that 25 percent of employees said work is their main source of stress, and 40 percent described their job as very or extremely stressful.

Some relationships in life we can choose, but workplace relationships often are thrust upon us. Although people often make friends through work, they also have to deal with personalities that don't personally mesh. Not seeing eye-to-eye with co-workers — or even employers — can cause extreme stress on the job.

In working relationships, sometimes emotional detachment can be the healthiest strategy for survival, according to Ann Michael, a business consultant and author of the Manage to Change blog.

"Passion can make you too close to something. We all need to be able to step back and disconnect. In order to see flaws in the plan, respect the input of others and maintain an open mind, a little indifference can go a long way," Michael writes.

Indifference actually can help people cope with stress at work. Becoming less attached to work tasks can make it easier to deal with criticism and change. For workers who feel trapped in a situation with a demanding boss, removing ego from job assignments can be an excellent coping mechanism. Harsh critiques won't seem like personal attacks, and emotional neutrality will make it easier to have peace of mind outside of the workplace.

If you feel caught in a dead-end job that isn't satisfying but feel unable to move on (possibly because of the economy), bring passion to other areas of your life. Devote yourself to physical fitness or take art classes. On your own time, pursue interests that further your sense of well-being.

10.13

Man's best friend

Single-people households may be on the rise, but so is pet ownership. According to a survey by the American Pet Products Association, 39 percent of U.S. households own at least one dog and 33 percent of U.S. households own at least one cat. Although Americans may have less contact with other humans than in the past, they have a record amount of time spent with companion animals.

But are pets a healthy substitute for friends? Recent research has shown that relationships with animals actually can have similar positive effects to close friendships. A study in the *Journal of Personality and Social Psychology* reports that pets confer significant benefits to their owners. In an examination of 217 members of a single community, pet owners showed greater self-esteem, were in better physical shape, were less lonely, were more conscientious and socially outgoing and tended to have healthier relationships with humans. In fact, people surveyed said that their pets provided as much support as their family members, and many said they were closer to their pets that they are to other people.

Get the notion of crazy cat ladies out of your head. The research actually found that most people do not turn to pets because their human social interaction is poor. Actually, pet owners seem to interact with their pets on the same level as they associate with other humans. Introverts and narcissists, for example, actually are less likely to report having positive experiences with pets. An individual who describes himself as a "people person" actually can find more value in pet ownership, according to the study.

Dogs aren't necessarily man's best friend, either. Researchers have found that any pet can have the same benefits. Pet owners of dogs, cats, horses, lizards, snakes and even fish all reported positive interactions.

A bond with animals can strengthen human resilience through moments of crises, adversity and disruptive transitions, including relocation, divorce, widowhood and adoption. Activities like petting a dog, for example, can cause a person's blood pressure to drop. The health benefits are even more significant. Patients who have a heart attack and own pets have five times the survival rate of patients who are not pet owners, according to the book *Heart Sense for Women* by cardiologist Stephen Sinatra. The National Center for Infectious Disease reports that pet ownership can decrease blood pressure, cholesterol levels and triglyceride levels. People who own pets also are more likely to exercise and socialize, according to the report.

The joy that pets bring humans might actually have a physiological explanation. A study by the Research Center for Human/Animal Interaction at the University of Missouri College of Veterinary Medicine found that interacting with animals increases the level of the hormone oxytocin, which helps us feel happy and trusting. The chemical reaction also may have more long-term significance.

"Oxytocin has some powerful effects for us in the body's ability to be in a state of readiness to heal and also to grow new cells, so it predisposes us to an environment in our bodies where we can be healthier," said Rebecca Johnson, a nurse who headed up the research.

"The eyes of my eyes are opened."
— *e.e. cummings*

CHAPTER **11.** Spirituality

"This is my simple religion.
There is no need for temples;
no need for complicated philosophy.
Our own brain, our own heart is our temple;
the philosophy is kindness."
— *Dalai Lama*

Wellness Wake-up Call

What is your biggest regret? It probably has little to do with possessions like cars or homes. At our core, humans value relationships with other humans. But quality relationships are even harder to acquire than a McMansion or Mercedes-Benz. Friendship and love require painful work — and forgiveness. How many people do you need to forgive?

Do you hold onto painful moments from your childhood? Has your relationship with your spouse suffered because of a past event that you can't let go? Do you maintain a grudge against a former friend for a perceived wrong? Do you lose sleep thinking about the people who were once meaningful in your life but have now become strangers — and the incidents that put a wedge between you? If you answered yes to any of these questions, that's a Wellness Wake-up Call...

11.2 Higher power

Ancient religious literature — including Christian, Hebrew, Buddhist, Confucian, Muslim and Hindu — all place emphasis on the power of forgiving. Forgiveness isn't about justice or being fair. In fact, it often is the complete opposite. To forgive someone, you have to recognize that you have been treated unjustly, then abandon resentment for the transgression. Forgiveness is no easy task, however. Most Americans value strength and a moral sense of what is right and wrong. In a culture that focuses on power and personal achievement, forgiveness often is viewed as a sign of weakness — as if in a dispute between two opponents, the forgiver bowed his head in submission.

Forgiveness, however, is far more difficult than resentment. Healthy relationships don't focus on who has the upper hand. Every relationship requires forgiveness to maintain itself, and forgiving someone requires you to let go of pain. Although you may not condone, excuse, or forget what happened, you choose not to let it continue to negatively affect you.

According to Dr. Mark Banschick in a Psychology Today article, forgiveness has a healing power that allows people to move on with their lives. But it is more than acceptance, which is essentially passive.

Forgiving someone requires conscious change. "Some people never forgive and never forget," Banschick writes. "They remain victims forever, not just victims of the insult that happened, but also to an identification with their wound that may have impact on future relationships and their sense of identity." Psychotherapist Frank Luskin, director of the Stanford University Forgiveness Project, notes how resentment can be a vicious cycle. "If you've been dumped or treated badly, and you don't really heal, you're going to be less trusting, more defensive, and more quarrelsome with the next guy — or even the next five — because you still carry visceral pain. When we can't move past that, we stay a prisoner of our worst experiences," Luskin said. While resentment is a weight that grows heavier and heavier, forgiveness enables freedom and growth.

11.3

Forgiveness times three

When people think of forgiveness, the first thing that comes to mind usually involves the wrongs others have done to us. But forgiveness actually has three forms. In addition to feeling the need to forgive others for their transgressions, seeking forgiveness for the things you have done can be equally important. A crucial part of the 12 steps recovery program of Alcoholics Anonymous involves admitting the nature of wrongs and making amends to the people who have been hurt.

In fact, the need to be accepted and forgiven is engrained in our DNA. Mark Leary, a psychologist at Duke University, claims that seeking forgiveness is part of human evolution. "Unlike virtually every other species, the hominids could not rely on speed, flight, strength, arboreal clambering, burrowing or ferocity to evade predators. Many theorists in psychology, anthropology and biology have noted that human beings and their hominid ancestors survived and prospered as species only because they lived in cooperative groups," Leary writes. "Given the importance of group living, natural selection favored individuals who not only sought the company of others but also behaved in ways that led others to accept, support and help them."

According to Leary, years of experiments conducted in social psychology indicate that individuals are more dependent on one another than we like to believe. Leary's sociometer showed that our self-esteem has as much to do with our connection to other people than it does to an inner force. Leary's research claims that statements like "it doesn't matter what anyone else says" have little validity in modern culture. Humans by nature need to be forgiven for the wrongs they commit against one another — so they can remain a valued part of the group.

Perhaps the hardest forgiveness of all is letting go of resentment for your own wrongs or perceived failures. Guilt and shame, even from childhood events, can linger through a lifetime. Self-forgiveness may be the most difficult — and most important — form of healing. "The human mind is sometimes an instrument of misery," said Loren Toussaint, a psychologist at Luther University in Iowa studying how forgiveness is linked to health. ""When you've done wrong to others and regret it, it bubbles up again and again. There's no escaping the perpetrator."

11.4

Scale of justice

Most people consider themselves to be fairly forgiving. Yet, if you truly look at your life, it's not hard to find times where forgiveness wasn't so easy. Whether you held a grudge for something small, like a missed lunch date, or couldn't let go of great pain from a significant event, like a car accident, resentment can be consuming like a cancer.

Although forgiveness seems like something intangible, researchers at the John Templeton Foundation developed a series of questions to measure an individuals' level of negativity — for ourselves, others and specific events. Asking respondents to answer with a range between "almost always false of me" and "almost always true of me," the Heartland Forgiveness Scale can help people recognize their own emotional baggage.

How forgiving are you? Are past wounds affecting your future?

Consider how you would respond to this sampling from the test

Almost always false of me — — — — — — — — — — — — — Almost always true of me

I hold grudges against myself for negative things I have done.

I continue to punish a person who has done something I think is wrong.

Although others have hurt me in the past, I eventually have been able to see them as good people.

When things go wrong for reasons that can't be controlled, I get stuck in negative thoughts about it.

It's really hard for me to accept negative situations that aren't anybody's fault.

11.5

Americans and forgiveness

Percentage of U.S. adults who report high levels of four types of forgiveness

Age in years:	18-44	45-64	65+
Forgiveness of self	53	62	59
Forgiveness of others	46	57	62
Forgiveness by God	69	80	79
Proactive Forgiveness	40	47	47

Percentage of U.S. men and women reporting high levels of forgiveness

	Men	Women
Forgiveness of self	56	57
Forgiveness of others	49	54
Forgiveness by God	71	77
Proactive Forgiveness	37	48

Source: University of Michigan Institute for Social Research 2001

"People are often unreasonable and self-centered.
Forgive them anyway. If you are kind,
people may accuse you of ulterior motives.
Be kind anyway. If you are honest,
people may cheat you. Be honest anyway.
If you find happiness, people may be jealous.
Be happy anyway. The good you do today may
be forgotten tomorrow. Do good anyway.
Give the world the best you have
and it may never be enough. Give your best anyway.
For you see, in the end, it is between you and God.
It was never between you and them anyway."

—*Mother Teresa*

11.6

Going through a stage

Don't think of forgiveness as a black-and-white issue. Like most emotional things, forgiveness is a process — and it can take time. The late psychiatrist Elizabeth Kubler-Roth, author of the classic book *On Death and Dying*, outlined the stages of grief, which include denial, bargaining, anger, depression and acceptance. In many ways, forgiveness is a sibling of grief that follows a similar cycle.

Psychologist Robert Enright has become an ambassador of forgiveness, even taking the strategies he developed for the book *The Forgiving Life* to Liberia to help its residents deal with the emotions of a long civil war. Enright acknowledges four stages of forgiveness — uncovering, decision, work and deepening.

Uncovering involves confronting anger and shame and gaining insight into what really happened. The step requires a person to look at how the event truly affected him or her. The *Decision* stage is about making choices, specifically accepting the real meaning of forgiveness and committing to the process of healing. Of course, the stages require work, which can include empathy and compassion. The person who feels wronged must gain a deeper understanding of his or her offender and begin to view the perpetrator in a different light. *Work* is not without pain, but it can lead to *deepening*, which allows for post-suffering growth. In the final stage, people discover that the process of forgiveness actually can help them feel more connected to others and decrease overall negative emotions.

The third stage — work — may be the most significant. Rudolf Klimes, author of the book *Spiritual Disorders* and founder of a continuing education program for health care professionals, breaks the forgiveness process into five steps. Instead of choosing on an eye for an eye, Klimes bases his process on Christian religious principles, including the philosophy of being kind to one another.

11.7   Steps to forgiveness

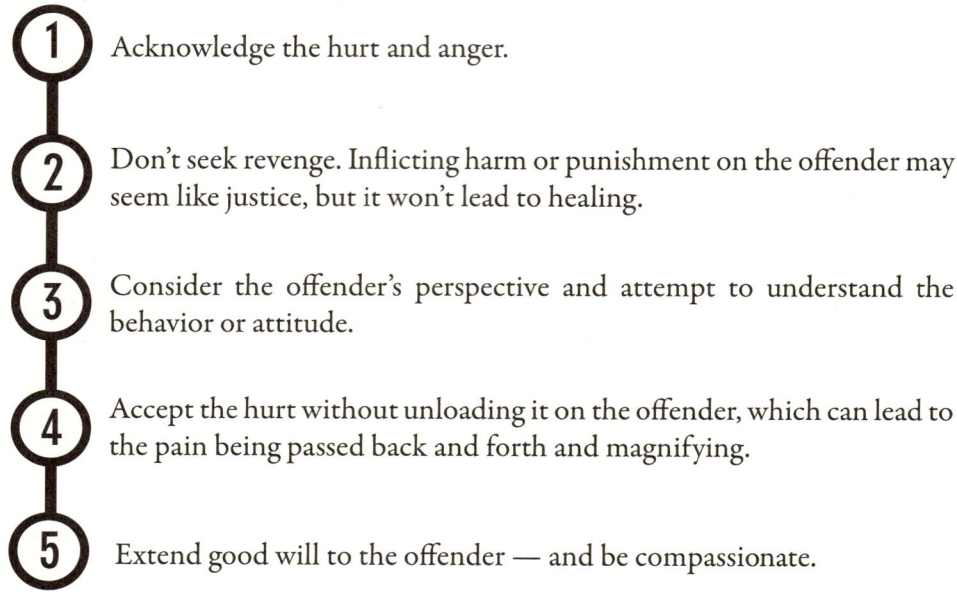

1 Acknowledge the hurt and anger.

2 Don't seek revenge. Inflicting harm or punishment on the offender may seem like justice, but it won't lead to healing.

3 Consider the offender's perspective and attempt to understand the behavior or attitude.

4 Accept the hurt without unloading it on the offender, which can lead to the pain being passed back and forth and magnifying.

5 Extend good will to the offender — and be compassionate.

11.8   Forgiveness with benefits

Forgiveness may seem like an abstract, but the process actually has measurable benefits. According to the Mayo Clinic, people who have learned to forgive have healthier relationships, greater spiritual and psychological well-being, less anxiety and hostility, better overall physical health, fewer symptoms of depression, and a lower risk of alcohol and substance abuse.

Think about someone you haven't forgiven for wronging you in the past. According to Luskin of the Stanford University Forgiveness Project, your body has a physical response. "When you think about a wrong someone did to you, your fight-or-flight system is aroused," Luskin said. "Your heart beats faster. Your blood pressure goes up. You feel hurt and mad. But you could be sitting here feeling how good it is to be alive on such a beautiful day. You won't always be alive, you know. So doesn't it

make more sense to appreciate this moment, this now?"
A recent field of research is uncovering direct correlations to unresolved interpersonal anger and poor health. Scientists have recorded a link to forgiveness and better immune functioning, less physiological reactivity to stress, lower blood pressure, and stronger mental health.

While resentment has been linked to high blood pressure and cardiopulmonary disease, forgiveness actually has been scientifically connected to recovery from a heart attack. Dr. Douglas Russell, a Veterans Health Administration cardiologist, reported an improvement in the coronary function of heart attack patients who had taken part in a 10-hour course in forgiveness.

Laura Kubzansky, an associate professor of society, human development and health at the Harvard School of Public Health, cites a number of findings that link positive actions, like forgiveness, to health. According to Kubzansky, individuals with emotional vitality have a 20 percent reduced risk of heart disease and highly optimistic people have half the risk of getting cardiovascular disease compared to their pessimistic counterparts.

A University of Michigan School of Public Health study found that married couples who felt free to express their feelings lived longer than those who were resentful of each other. The research followed 192 couples in a small Michigan town over 17 years. Twenty-six of the couples consisted of relationships where both spouses developed resentment and failed to resolve problems. These couples showed significantly higher death rates. In the 26 pairs, 13 deaths were reported. In the remaining 166 couples, only 41 deaths occurred. In the angry couples, both spouses died in 23 percent of the pairs, versus 6 percent in the more emotionally healthy marriages. "I suspect that forgiveness may prove to be a sort of psychological antidote to anger, which has already shown to have a host of negative physical and mental health effects," said Loren Toussaint, who conducted a study for the Institute for Social Research.

Much like nutrition and exercise, forgiveness should be an important part of every health regimen. And like other healthy choices, it's never too late to start.

"The weak can never forgive.
Forgiveness is the attribute of the strong."
— *Gandhi*

11.9

Going through the motions

There is more to forgiveness than simply saying, I'm sorry. We all can remember childhood fights where our parents forced us to issue an insincere apology to someone we had wronged. Although the parental gesture was meant to be positive, in reality, the coerced statement of apology had little effect.

Forgiveness requires sincerity — whether you are seeking someone's absolution, forgiving someone who has done something wrong to you or allowing yourself to heal from past mistakes. Fake forgiveness is as detrimental as no forgiveness at all. Jeanne Safer, a New York psychoanalyst, is the author of *Must We Forgive?* In the book, Safer argues that forgiveness may not be possible for everyone — or at least may take longer to achieve. "For many patients, forgiveness is a double whammy: First someone screws you, and then it's your fault you don't want to embrace them in heaven. I'm not against forgiveness. I'm against compulsory forgiveness with no choice," Safer states. "And I'm against 'forgiveness lite,' which keeps you from feeling the intensity of the experience, from deeply grappling with what's been done to you."

Safer's real fear is that victims will turn a fake forgiveness into self-blame. Research by Lydia Temoshok, a clinical and social psychologist at the University of Maryland's Institute of Human Virology, noticed a link between self-blamers and health. Looking at patients infected with the HIV virus, those who tended to deny problems, suppress strong feelings and remain in stressful situations suffered greater complications form the disease. According to Temoshok, people who are in denial about their feelings are more likely to have the HIV virus progress to AIDS, as well as see the progression of melanoma. To quote a classic Elton John song, "Sorry seems to be the hardest word."

"I have learned that sometimes "sorry" is not enough.
Sometimes you actually have to change."
— *Claire London*

11.10

Amazing grace

Roman Catholics go to confession to seek absolution from their sins. Yom Kippur, the holiest day of the year for Jewish people, is a 24-hour period of fasting and intensive prayer for atonement. The followers of Islam not only seek the forgiveness of Allah through repentance, but they also believe it is important for humans to both forgive and be forgiven. Forgiveness is a common thread in all of the major religions, and all faiths have structures that allow followers to connect to each other and the world. Through an organized belief system, cultural links, world views, moral codes, and spirituality, each religion provides important support to its congregation members.

A new field of science has begun to study how faith is connected to health. In the book *The Longevity Project,* Howard S. Friedman and Leslie Martin examine the habits and careers of more than 1,500 California residents who were first studied as children in 1921. In addition to a number of other topics, the subjects reported on their religious instruction, worship, Bible reading, and levels of faith at points throughout their lives. Looking through eight decades of data, the authors noticed some interesting correlations between religious worship and life spans. The findings indicated that people who were religious, especially women, were more likely to live longer lives. On the other hand, the women in the study who were the least religious, on average, had shorter life spans, and people who let their religious involvement wane were at high risk of earlier mortality, especially if they also let their community involvement decrease. But the authors don't necessarily attribute the longevity of the devout to divine intervention. Instead, they found that religious women tended to be friendly and sociable and maintained strong social ties and healthy behaviors. *The Longevity Project* did uncover good evidence that at least some aspects of congregational participation can be relevant to the length of one's mortal life," Friedman states.

Similarly, a project by Neal Krause of the University of Michigan showed that people who received social support for stress through their church report themselves to be healthier than people who receive similar support from secular sources.

According to Dr. Harold Koenig, the director of Duke University's Center for Spirituality, Theology and Health, research indicates that people who are religious are more physically active and take better care of themselves. They live longer, have fewer heart attacks, are less likely to be depressed and more likely to feel like their life has significance.

A study of 179 patients who had received a liver transplant showed a connection between people who believed in a higher power and a more successful recovery. The report, published in the journal Liver Transplantation, found that those who were actively seeking God, despite their particular branch of faith, had a better survival rate, as opposed to patients who reported no religious beliefs at all. In fact some patients were up to three times more likely to survive, even if they didn't attend church but claimed to have a strong religious connection. "We found that an active search for God (where) the patient's faith in a higher power rather than a generic destiny, had a positive impact on patient survival," said Dr. Franco Bonaguido, leader of the study. Two years after the transplants, religious patients were three times more likely to survive. After three years, more than 20 percent of the non-religious patients had died, while only about 7 percent of the actively seeking God patients had passed away.

A growing number of medical facilities and hospitals are taking notice of the growing research on religion and health. Duke University, the University of Florida, the University of Minnesota and other institutions have created academic centers dedicated to the study of religion and medicine, and around 66 percent of medical schools across the country now offer classes on spirituality and health (that number was only 2 percent in the 1990s) — and 75 percent of the schools that offer the classes consider the training to be mandatory. "There's been a sea change in the way the medical community looks at spirituality," said Dr. Christina Puchalski, an internist who founded the George Washington University Institute for Spirituality and Health.

"Unitas, veritas and caritas." (community, truth, and love)
— *St. Augustine*

> "If the only prayer you ever say in your entire life is thank you, it will be enough."
> — *Meister Eckhart*

11.11   Gratitude

Gratitude is a common tenet around the world in Christianity, Islam, Buddhism, Judaism and Hinduism. It is also, as research increasingly shows, an important and basic part of living a happy life.

According to a 2003 study by Robert Emmons and Michael McCullough, those who kept gratitude journals on a weekly basis did all sort of healthy actions more than those who didn't keep the gratitude journals. They "exercised more regularly, reported fewer physical symptoms, felt better about their lives as a whole and were more optimistic about the upcoming week compared to those who recorded hassles or neutral life events."

Hold your own gratitude intervention

Take two minutes and find a quiet corner. Close your eyes and start silently considering your gratitude list of the day. You're encouraged to list the biggies — for example, parents who loved you and did their best — to the small things in life that brighten your day or make you smile — orange juice with no pulp, maybe. Big or small, for two minutes, consider the people, their actions and things that you choose to add to your gratitude list.

Another option is to create your own gratitude ritual — every time you're stopped at a red light, for example.

Beyond the positive actions, the people who kept gratitude journals were also "more likely to have made progress toward important personal goals," — including academic, interpersonal and health-based, according to highlights of the research project by Emmons and McCullough.

Some facts from the study of those who kept gratitude journals

16 percent fewer physical symptoms.

19 percent more time exercising.

10 percent less physical pain.

8 percent more sleep.

25 percent increased sleep quality.

The study revealed documented benefits of gratitude that didn't stop there. Young adults who participated in daily gratitude interventions reported higher "levels of positive states of alertness, enthusiasm, determination, attentiveness and energy." In general, the study concluded that grateful people seem to be happier overall, certainly with a brighter attitude toward the future. They reported "higher levels of life satisfaction, vitality, optimism and lower levels of depression and stress," according to the study. In fact, the "disposition toward gratitude appears to enhance pleasant feeling states more than it diminishes unpleasant emotions. Grateful people do not deny or ignore the negative aspects of life."

In a 2002 study by McCullough, Emmons and Tsang, those with a strong disposition toward gratitude were shown to have more capacity toward empathy and try to see another person's perspective than those with a lower disposition toward gratitude. Additionally, grateful people are more likely to be more spiritual and "acknowledge a belief in the interconnectedness of all life and a commitment to and responsibility to others."

When it comes to materialism, grateful individuals would have scored high marks on a kindergarten report card. They were shown to "place less importance on material goods; they are less likely to judge their own and others success in terms of possessions accumulated; they are less envious of others; and are more likely to share their possessions with others relative to less grateful persons."

> "Reflect on your present blessings,
> on which every man has many,
> not on your past misfortunes,
> of which all men have some."
> — *Charles Dickens*

11.12 The many benefits of gratitude

Research shows that, overall, being grateful can lead to more happiness than winning the lottery. And if that's not enough, being grateful does a whole lot more.

- Gratitude makes you sleep better.
- Gratitude leads to more exercise.
- Gratitude strengthens physiological functioning and leads to improved health.
- Gratitude leads to feeling better.
- Gratitude makes you friendlier.
- Gratitude helps you get along with others better.
- Gratitude diminishes the green monster of envy.
- Gratitude leads to better relationships, including a happier marriage.
- Gratitude makes you a better manager at work.
- Gratitude improves decision-making.
- Gratitude makes you more productive.

11.13   A spirited conversation

Although spirituality is at the core of all major religions, people don't have to follow a specific religion or attend a house of worship to be spiritual — and spiritual people also fare well in health statistics. Spirituality isn't about a prescribed dogma. Spiritual people may be religious, but they also feel a connection to the world and other people. They are self-aware. Rather than living by hard and fast rules, they aspire toward perfection, beauty and enlightenment. Spirituality is a journey rather than a doctrine that can be studied in a book.

Becoming a more spiritual person can help relieve stress, which can lead to a healthier life. It also can give you a greater sense of purpose by clarifying what is most important to you. Through the process, you will feel a greater connection to the world, which in turn can give you a better sense of self-worth. Spirituality allows people to release control, which makes it easier to share both the happy and difficult times in life with others. The greater connectivity will expand your support network, whether it be through joining a religious congregation or reaching out to family and friends.

> "Gratitude is not only the greatest of virtues,
> but the parent of all the others."
> —*Cicero*

11.14   Spirituality requires inward reflection

To work on your own spirituality, consider the following questions:

- What are my most important relationships?
- What do I value most in life?
- What people give me a sense of community?
- What inspires me and gives me hope?
- What makes me happy?
- What are my proudest achievements?

11.15

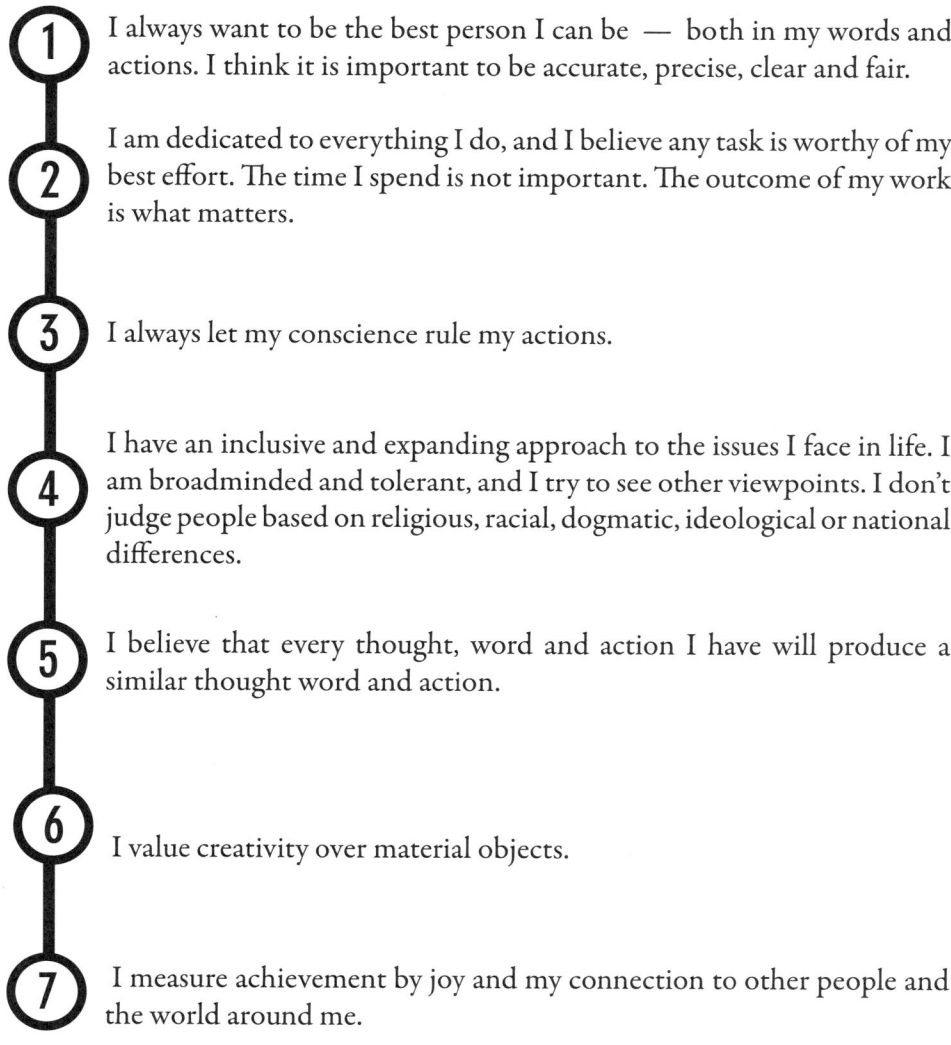

1   I always want to be the best person I can be — both in my words and actions. I think it is important to be accurate, precise, clear and fair.

2   I am dedicated to everything I do, and I believe any task is worthy of my best effort. The time I spend is not important. The outcome of my work is what matters.

3   I always let my conscience rule my actions.

4   I have an inclusive and expanding approach to the issues I face in life. I am broadminded and tolerant, and I try to see other viewpoints. I don't judge people based on religious, racial, dogmatic, ideological or national differences.

5   I believe that every thought, word and action I have will produce a similar thought word and action.

6   I value creativity over material objects.

7   I measure achievement by joy and my connection to other people and the world around me.

(If all of the above statements describe you, then you are on a spiritual path. Statements that don't match are areas you might want to evaluate.)

11.16

Like a prayer

Prayer is a crucial component in the benefits of religion and spirituality, according to a number of research reports. But prayer is more than just reciting a memorized text, like a *Hail Mary*, with little thought. To be effective, prayer must involve reflection and an outpouring of emotion.

Using electronic imaging technology, Andrew Newberg of the University of Pennsylvania analyzed the brain waves of a group of nuns as they prayed. The results showed a more complicated functioning than seen during many other activities. While praying, the nuns had increased levels of activity in the frontal lobes, which corresponds with concentration. But they also had changes in the brain regions related to emotion, behavior, long-term memory and the sense of self. According to Newberg, few other tasks show such a complex level of activity. Prayer can take many forms. Christians may bow their heads, fold their hands and kneel, while many American Indian tribes consider dancing as a connection to a higher power. A Hindu might chant a mantra, and many followers of Islam whirl as a form of meditation. At Quaker meetings, congregation members practice silent prayer.

But prayer doesn't have to be an organized activity. A walk in the woods or personal moment of reflection also can be considered a form of prayer. The most important component of prayer, however, is sincerity. Simply going through the motions has little effect.

One research study that examined 1,800 patients recovering from cardiac surgery found that although prayer can have positive health effects on people who pray, intercessory prayer (prayers by other people for someone else's welfare) did nothing to help patients heal. A group of around 600 patients who unknowingly received prayer had similar survival rates to another group of 600 that didn't receive prayer. Oddly, a third group of patients who knew they were receiving prayers actually fared worse.

The benefits of prayer and spirituality are personal. In many ways, prayer is like the homework on the path to enlightenment. But you have to do it yourself.

"If you have accomplished all that
you have planned for yourself,
you have not planned enough."
—Edward Everett

CHAPTER 12. Maintenance

Wellness Wake-up Call

Have you started an exercise program that gave you the results you're looking for originally, but your results have tapered off? Are you frustrated with where you are because you're no longer getting the results you were?

This is a Wellness Wake-up Call.

12.2

Owning a home has become a standard part of the American Dream — and for most homeowners, that purchase is looked at as a long-term investment. It's a major expenditure that is expected to build equity over time. Our house is our fortress — a castle where all the great memories of life unfold.

But homeownership requires more than just writing a month check to the mortgage company. Dream homes are filled with responsibility. Whether you purchase a fixer-upper that demands endless renovations or a new McMansion that is the envy of the neighborhood, houses require daily maintenance. The lawn needs to be mowed and the garden requires weeding. You have to wash windows and scrub floors. Over time, signs of wear need to be spruced up. You paint the trim, remodel the kitchen and upgrade the bathroom. You try to prevent slight problems from becoming big emergencies. If the roof starts to leak, you don't want to just do a stop-gap shingle patch. You want to protect your investment from future damage.

Homeownership is a commitment that is both frustrating and rewarding. The more effort you put into your home, the more you get back. Hard work turns a house into a home. You want your neighbors to notice its curb appeal and expect that it is a reflection of what is inside.

For some reason, most Americans don't apply the same principles to their bodies, which really are the true home where we live. Like a piece of valuable real estate, our bodies are a long-term investment that requires maintenance. The more work you do, the better the return on your investment. Just like you can't slap a coat of paint on a crumbling wall, our bodies require more than just cosmetic attention. Health is about building a strong foundation and continuing to do work every day to maintain and improve.

How many people do you know who have gone on diets and hit the gym when they decided they wanted to lose 20 pounds? In a few months, they reach their weight goal. They look better, and their self-esteem gets a boost. But then they drop the healthier habits they developed to reach that goal. They start eating fast food at lunch, skip the workouts and spend evenings back on the couch. Soon, they gain back the 20 pounds — or more — and feel even worse about themselves.

Good health isn't a rental agreement. It's a long-term mortgage. Keeping our foundations solid is the key to living a long and happy existence. This book isn't about quick fixes. It's about changing bad habits, adopting a healthy lifestyle and maintaining exercise and proper nutrition for the rest of your life.

12.3 Hard habit to break

What are your worst habits? Do you crave cupcakes or bags of tortilla chips? Do you smoke? Would you rather sit on the couch watching marathons of reality television rather than get up and jog around the block? That sensation that keeps you committed to your old, unhealthy self is the result of myelin.

Remember myelination, the physiological process that turns our behavior patterns — both good and bad — into roadmaps for the future? All of those negative habits you have continue to tempt you because of myelin. But you can turn the tables. As previously discussed, the same myelin that makes it difficult for us to correct negative behavior also can set us on a healthier path. It might feel like you are changing the course of a raging river, but once you switch directions, you'll find yourself in an easier flow.

"Habits play an important role in our health," said Dr. Nora Volkow, director of the National Institute of Health's drug abuse sector. "Understanding the biology of how we develop routines that may be harmful to us, and how to break those routines and embrace new ones, could help us change our lifestyles and adopt healthier behaviors."

Heidi Grant Halvorson, a social psychologist and author of *Succeed: How We Can Reach Our Goals*, suggests that there actually is a scientific method to breaking bad habits to bring positive change into our lives.

According to Halvorson, the first step is to identify the problem. Where most people fail in this stage is that they aren't specific. For example, it's not enough to say, "I want to exercise more." To effectively change a habit, you have to set measurable goals. Give yourself a standard. "I want to walk for 30 minutes five days a week" is a goal you can assess on a daily basis. You can hold yourself accountable and make specific changes to negative patterns.

Nothing worthwhile is easy. Acknowledge that attaining your new goal is going to be difficult. You can quit smoking, but it won't be easy.

Halvorson notes that people who are realistic about the challenges they face are more likely to plan, put forth greater effort, and tend to be more persistent. If you expect to work hard, you will work hard. A study of women going through a weight-loss program found that the participants who expected dieting to be hard actually had better results. The women who acknowledged that resisting the temptation of junk food would be difficult lost 24 more pounds than the participants who expected that it would be easy to resist sweets and snack foods. The woman who knew they were facing a difficult process went out of their way to avoid temptation — and they were more successful as a result.

One of the real keys of breaking bad habits is to have a clear understanding of your own willpower. Halvorson likens willpower to a muscle — our capacity for self-control grows stronger with regular exercise. But just as your muscles get fatigued after a good workout, your willpower can weaken when you've had a particularly stressful day. When you feel drained and vulnerable, be prepared in advance. If you don't have the energy to run, try walking as an alternative exercise. If you know you might crave a bucket of popcorn at the end of the day, make sure you have healthier snack alternatives on hand instead.

Although we may feel like creatures of habit, humans actually have an advantage over other animals — our brains are wired to make change easier. "Humans are much better than any other animal at changing and orienting our behavior toward long-term goals, or long-term benefits," said Roy Baumeister, a Florida State University psychologist. "We've found that you can improve your self control by doing exercise over time. Any regular act of self control will gradually exercise your 'muscle' and make you stronger."

And don't forget, change is a process. It's not going to happen overnight. Celebrate the victories you do make. When you find yourself attaining a positive goal, reward yourself with a healthy treat — like a massage or a new article of clothing.

Turning bad habits into positive behavior isn't just a temporary exercise. Make healthy lifestyle choices, and maintain them over time. It won't be easy — and there will be plenty of temptations along the way — but the benefits of success will far outweigh any difficulties you encountered along the way.

12.4

Ch-ch-changes

If only there were a magic machine we could get on and it would magically make us fit.

Although infomercials make ab blasters and all-over body workout equipment seem like quick solutions to our fitness ills, there isn't one machine that can help you maintain your fitness level over time.

If you are just starting an exercise program or want to ramp up your routine, think health instead of weight loss or body image. Although looking better is a great result of exercise, it shouldn't be the primary goal. If you focus on being healthier instead, you're more likely to stick with your new lifestyle over time. People who begin to exercise because they want to drop a few pounds tend to get discouraged more easily. They also often go back to inactivity once they've shed the pounds.

Keeping a written log of your exercise will have you stay on track and also show you any pitfalls you may encounter along the way. Set a goal, say riding a stationary bike for 30 minutes for five days a week, and then mark your actual session on a calendar. If you falter for a week, analyze why you didn't meet your goal. Is your evening schedule too hectic and therefore you need to get up 30 minutes earlier to find the time for exercise? Are you bored by the activity and need to find something else to hold your interest? Are you just making excuses? Be honest with yourself. This is about your life, and you need to take control and assume responsibility for your healthier future.

If exercise seems boring, think of ways you could make it more entertaining. Get one of your friends to become a workout buddy, and make a pact to be supportive of each other's goals. Going to the gym with a friend can become a pleasant social activity and it may help break the monotony. Another way to make exercise more enjoyable — and therefore more likely to become part of your daily routine — is to incorporate music. Whether you listen to your favorite tunes on your iPod while jogging on a treadmill or take an aerobic dance class, music can make the time pleasurable rather than just a chore.

Some days motivation will be more difficult than others. Set a minimum standard for yourself, then push yourself to go further. Mentally divide your workout routine into chunks. On those first seconds on the elliptical machine, it's easier to think about completing 15 minutes than it is an hour. Give yourself the option of stopping at this point, but encourage yourself to persist for a second 15 minute segment. At each check point, mentally reward yourself for your commitment and endurance. Psychologically, the workout will feel more like a challenge than an insurmountable task.

Even professional athletes get in exercise ruts. Although it is important to make exercise a part of your regular routine, working out requires challenging our bodies. Walking on a treadmill for 30 minutes might be effective when you first start a regimen, but your body will adapt to the activity. Soon it will become second nature — and you won't see the same fitness results.

After a month of consistent aerobic activity, you will be a different person. Your fitness level will change, and you have to change your routine along with it.

Just as our minds might get bored by repeating the same activities day after day, so do our bodies. If you don't vary your fitness routine, you eventually will plateau. You can continue to do the same exercise program that got you amazing results for several weeks, and suddenly you feel stuck. You're not losing weight and you don't see any other signs of improving your health. Your body is in a rut.

Variety is more than just the spice of life, it's an essential element to successful workouts. Your body needs to be challenged, and your exercise program needs to evolve. If you consistently change your workout, your body won't adapt — and you'll see better results. Athletes often use periodization, a planned training progression, to avoid hitting a plateau.

When working with athletes, some fitness experts will break the year up into three cycles: one focusing on strength, one on endurance and another on speed and muscle tone. Another common approach is to increase the intensity of workouts. Even if you continue to exercise for 30 minutes, change the order and type of exercises you perform. For example, if you are doing weight training with bench presses, try switching to push-ups or dumbbell presses instead. On the stair climber, try adding four-minute bursts where you increase the speed, then adjust the intensity back down to your standard pace.

Another option is to rotate the gym equipment you use, switch between the treadmill and the elliptical machine. Although most people don't like change, our bodies crave it when it comes to improving our fitness levels.

12.5

Scales of justice

America is a nation of dieters. We eat poorly, gain excess weight, then fight to lose it. Once we've dropped a few pounds, most of us repeat the vicious cycle.

Although losing weight can be difficult, keeping the pounds off seems to be the bigger struggle. Successful weight maintenance requires regular exercise, smart dietary choices and constant monitoring. Fitness is a commitment.

Most dieters are very conscious of the scale, noting weight loss from week to week with bated breath. But once the extra pounds are gone, they put away the scale. Suddenly, accountability and measures no longer exist. According to a number of research studies, people who weigh themselves at least once a week are more successful in keeping off the pounds. It's better to detect small weight gains when they can easily be corrected then to suddenly notice 10 pounds of extra fat two weeks before your 25th high school reunion. The same food guidelines used to lose weight should apply to daily life. Eating is about health first and pleasure second. Make choices based on what will give your body the most energy rather than what foods set off positive triggers in your brain's reward center. Retrain your mind to crave fruit over cookies.

Keeping a food journal of everything you eat and drink is a common weight-loss tactic, but it also works well for people who want to maintain their weight. By adding accountability to your diet, it becomes more difficult to cheat. What you put in your mouth is laid out in front of you in black and white.

When you do falter, make a note of the situation. Emotional triggers often drive people back to unhealthy junk food. Identify these traps and avoid them. If being alone in your house makes you feel lonely and therefore crave high-fat food, try to become more social. Get a group of your friends together. Go out for a walk or volunteer for a local nonprofit group. Replacing a negative with a positive behavior is a great way to change bad habits that can become fitness stumbling blocks.

Understanding the psychology of weight gain can be as important as knowing the physiology. Most people know that high-fat foods are unhealthy but have become conditioned to make bad choices. Retraining your mind will change your waistline.

Holidays are a common trigger for many people. Most of the foods we associate with the season — from candied sweet potatoes to pies and cakes — are high in fat and sugar. Our subconscious minds correlate the happiness of the celebration with eating poorly, and we make unhealthy food choices out of habit.

Researchers used to believe that the average American gained about five pounds from November through December. A recent study has shown that number is actually not as significant. According to the National Institute of Health, Americans gain about one pound during the season. The problem comes from the fact that only a small percentage of those who gain weight lose the extra pound after the first of the new year. If that was the only pound you gained all year, that might not seem too extreme. But consider the situation over time. In a decade, you will have gained 10 pounds. Each year you gradually get heavier. Incremental small gains over time can lead to obesity.

A Stanford School of Medicine study found that mental preparation for weight loss is as important as dieting itself, especially when it comes to weight maintenance. Michael Kiernan, a senior research scientist at the Stanford Prevention Research Center, found that mastering weight-maintenance skills before even attempting to lose weight could achieve better results in the big picture. The research project divided a group of women who wanted to lose weight into two groups. The first set of women spent eight weeks mastering weight-maintenance techniques before taking on the task of actually losing weight. The second group focused on weight loss alone.

For frequent dieters, the results might be a little surprising. During the study period, the women who learned weight-maintenance before dieting lost the same amount of weight as the group that started dieting immediately. But more significant, the women who learned weight-maintenance skills had better results in keeping off the extra pounds. On average, they had regained three pounds a year after the study. The women who had jumped into dieting averaged a seven-pound gain.

"Those eight weeks were like a practice run," Kiernan said. "Women could try out different stability skills and work out the kinks without the pressure of worrying about how much weight they had lost. We found that waiting those eight weeks didn't make the women any less successful at losing weight. But even better, women who practiced stability first were more successful in maintaining that loss after a year."

12.6   Weight maintenance made easy

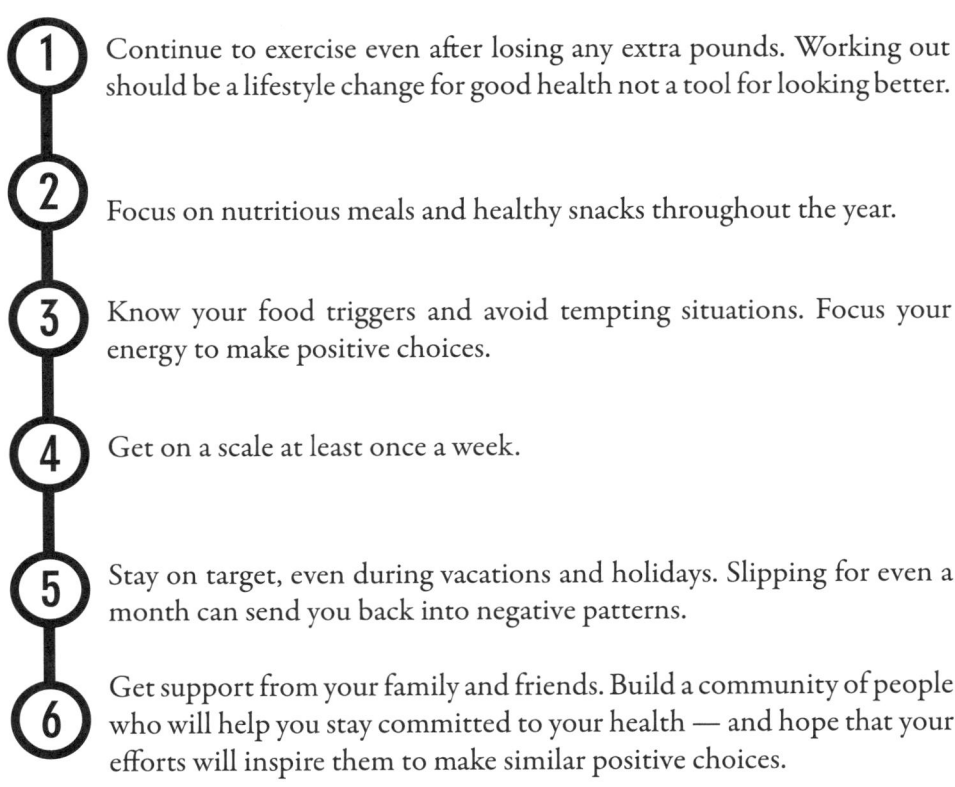

1 Continue to exercise even after losing any extra pounds. Working out should be a lifestyle change for good health not a tool for looking better.

2 Focus on nutritious meals and healthy snacks throughout the year.

3 Know your food triggers and avoid tempting situations. Focus your energy to make positive choices.

4 Get on a scale at least once a week.

5 Stay on target, even during vacations and holidays. Slipping for even a month can send you back into negative patterns.

6 Get support from your family and friends. Build a community of people who will help you stay committed to your health — and hope that your efforts will inspire them to make similar positive choices.

12.7   Go to the head of the class

By 2050, as many as 16 million Americans will be living with Alzheimer's disease, according to a report form the National Center for Chronic Disease Prevention and Health Promotion. The disease is now the sixth leading cause of death in adults and the fifth leading cause of death for people 65 and older.

Although the causes of Alzheimer's disease remain a mystery, diet is a key factor in prolonged brain health. The same healthy food choices that can prevent and control high blood pressure, diabetes, cardiovascular disease, obesity, and high cholesterol also are good for the brain. Just as obesity makes it difficult for people to walk, it also affects their brains. Eating low-fat food improves brain functions. In addition, antioxidants, which are known for fighting cancer, also neutralize harmful free radicals, which can benefit the brain.

The consumption of high doses of fish oil also can dramatically alter brain function, according to some researchers. The oils contain long-chain, omega-3 fatty acids that increase blood flow.

The brain is only about 2 percent of a person's total body mass, but the organ accounts for more than 25 percent of the blood flow. So, it makes sense that exercise is another key component to keeping your brain fit. Aerobic exercise increases capillary development in the brain, which means a greater access to blood, nutrients and oxygen. Some studies actually link regular workouts to improved brain health, and sedentary habits to mental decline.

But how do you know if your brain is at its peak efficiency? Mental fuzziness, jittery nerves, inability to focus on tasks and depression can all be signs of poor brain health. Ask yourself these questions:

- Do I have a hard time concentrating on my daily tasks?
- Do I move from project to project without completing the one at hand?
- Do I have a hard time getting organized?
- Do I have problems with my memory?
- Do I find it difficult to look forward to the future?
- Do I often feel sad?
- Do I feel hostile toward other people?

If you answered *yes* to any of the questions, your brain might need a boost, which should include better attention to diet and exercise. Your brain is like a computer's microprocessor that controls every function of your body. Brain health is crucial to your overall health. Never take this precious organ for granted.

12.8

50 ways to strain your brain

Try this. For the next 21 days try at least one of the following 50 activities. Keep a record of those you've tried. At the end of the three weeks, gauge your mood and energy level to note the difference.

☐ Do word puzzles, like scrabble or crosswords.
☐ Subscribe to a newspaper.
☐ Check out a classic novel from the library you've always meant to read.
☐ Work a jigsaw puzzle.
☐ Adopt a hobby that involves crafting or woodworking. Working with your hands also challenges the brain.
☐ Write letters or emails to friends on a regular basis.
☐ Rake the yard.
☐ Walk the dog.
☐ Go for a swim.
☐ Sign up for a yoga class.
☐ Look for a local park and take a hike.
☐ Join a dance class.
☐ Pick up an old sport you haven't played since high school.
☐ Take an adult learning class at a local college.
☐ Play a musical instrument.
☐ Join a choral group.
☐ Study a foreign language.
☐ Try doing tasks with your less dominant hand.
☐ Volunteer at a museum.
☐ Travel to new places.
☐ Eat more fish.
☐ Increase the amount of fruit and vegetables in your diet.
☐ Always eat breakfast.
☐ Drink green tea, which is rich in antioxidants.
☐ Stay hydrated. Drink two liters of water per day.
☐ Avoid fast food.
☐ Skip sugar for healthier snacks, like fruit.
☐ Reduce your caffeine intake.
☐ Keep alcohol consumption to a minimum.
☐ Get plenty of rest.
☐ Check your food labels; reduce your consumption of processed food.

☐ Try to stay away from pollutants, including toxins in cleaning products.

☐ Wear a helmet while riding a bike, skiing or rollerblading.

☐ Don't smoke.

☐ Prevent heat strokes by wearing a hat and staying hydrated.

☐ Be a safe driver.

☐ Use the handrails on steps and stairs to prevent injuries.

☐ Don't do recreational drugs, which can diminish brain capacity.

☐ Wear a seatbelt whenever you are in a car.

☐ Keep in touch with your emotions.

☐ Reduce stress in your life.

☐ Meditate.

☐ Say *yes* a little more often. Positivity is important.

☐ Get a pet.

☐ Attend a music concert.

☐ Call someone on the phone and have a conversation instead of sending a text message.

☐ Try an ethnic food you've never had before.

☐ Plant a garden.

☐ Be more loving and accepting.

☐ Don't take life too seriously.

12.9

Plan your future

Health doesn't come in a pill. Every day of your life should be committed to making the most of your health with positive lifestyle choices. Don't wait until you are sick to think about it.

Get off the couch. Clean out the kitchen cupboard of any processed food. Read a book. Go for a jog. Focus your attention on making good choices. You only have one life to live. It's never too late for a *Wellness Wake-up Call*.

"You can't build a reputation on what you're going to do."
—*Henry Ford*

BIBLIOGRAPHY

CHAPTER 1

Idaghdour, Youssef. . Genetic and Environmental Components of Human Leukocyte Gene Expression Variation in Morocco. (2009) Genetic and Environmental Components of Human Leukocyte Gene Expression Variation in Morocco. http://repository.lib.ncsu.edu/ir/bitstream/1840.16/5608/1/etd.pdf

CHAPTER 2

Society for Neuroscience (April 1, 2012) Critical Periods in Early Life. http://www.brainfacts.org/Brain-Basics/Brain-Development/Articles/2012/Critical-Periods-in-Early-Life

Brain Facts: A Primer on the Brain and Central Nervous System. (2012) Society for Neuroscience. p. 17. http://www.brainfacts.org/about-neuroscience/brain-facts-book/~/media/Brainfacts/Article%20Multimedia/About%20Neuroscience/Brain%20Facts%20book.ashx

Bartzokis George, Lu Po H, Geschwind Daniel H, Tingus Kathleen, Huang Danny, Mendez Mario F, Edwards Nancy, Mintz Jim (2007) Apolipoprotein E affects both myelin breakdown and cognition: implications for age-related trajectories of decline into dementia.. Biological psychiatry.

CHAPTER 3

Vlahos, James (2011, April 14). Is sitting a lethal activity? The New York Times. Retrieved from www.nytimes.com.

Center for Disease Control and Prevention (2003, Aug. 15). Prevalence of physical activity, including lifestyle activities among adults – United States, 2000-2001. Retrieved from www.cdc.gov.

Goodman, Brenda (2012, July 17). Sitting a lot can be 'very bad' for you. WebMD. Retrieved from www.webmd.com.

Reynolds, Gretchen (2012, April 28). Don't just sit there. The New York Times. Retrieved from www.nytimes.com.

Health Day (2012, April 7). Middle-age Americans less mobile than ever. Retrieved from www.healthday.com.

Seng, Raymond Lee Geok (undated). Inactivity speeds up aging. Retrieved from http://health.learninginfo.org.

CHAPTER 4

Science Daily (2007, May 11). Myelin. Retrieved from www.sciencedaily.com.

Greenfield, Ben (2011, May 30). How to exercise in the water. Quick and Dirty Tips. Retrieved from www.getfitguy.quickanddirtytips.com.

Chappell, Bill (2012, April 16). Americans do not walk the walk, and that's a growing problem. National Public Radio. Retrieved from www.npr.org.

Pool Corporation (2012). Benefits of exercising in water. Retrieved from www.swimmingpool.com.

Center for Disease Control and Prevention (2012, Feb. 24). Health benefits of water-based exercise. Retrieved from www.cdc.gov.

Ianzito, Christina (2011, March 24). The healing powers of dance. AARP Magazine. Retrieved from www.aarp.org.

Pizer, Ann (2012, Aug. 11). Yoga stretches at your desk. Retrieved from http://yoga.about.com.

Mayo Clinic (2010, Jan. 16). Yoga: Tap into the many health benefits. Retrieved from www.mayoclinic.com.

WebMD (undated). The health benefits of yoga. Retrieved from www.webmd.com.

U.S. News & World Report (2009, April 10). How to prevent falls by improving your balance. Retrieved from http://health.usnews.com.

Kouzmanoff, Abbie (2012, May 24). Study links consistent exercise and cognition. Dartmouth University. Retrieved from www.thedartmouth.com.

Grohol, John M. (2008, Jan. 10). The psychology of exercise and fitness. Psych Central. Retrieved from www.psychcentral.com.

Platkin, Charles Stuart (2008, August). Children's games that can help the whole family get in shape. Fitness Magazine. Retrieved from www.fitnessmagazine.com.

Hatfield, Heather (undated). WebMD Weight Loss Clinic. Retrieved from www.webmd.com.

Guilfot, Chrisitne (2009, Oct. 8). The important relationship between flexibility and health. Retrieved from www.medicalnewstoday.com.

Mayo Clinic (2011, Feb. 23). Stretching: Focus on flexibility. Retrieved from www.mayoclinic.com.

Mazzeo, Robert S. (undated). Exercise and the older adult. American College of Sports Medicine. Retrieved from www.acsm.org.

CHAPTER 5

Zeid, Elisa (2007, October 5). Some try extreme calorie restriction for long life. Msnbc.com. Retrieved from www.msnbc.com.

Szalavitz, Maia (2012, April 5). Can food really be addictive? Time, Healthland. Retrieved from http://healthland.time.com.

Klein, Sarah (2010, March 30). Fatty foods may cause cocaine-like addiction. Health. Retrieved from www.cnn.com.

Hatfield, Heather (2006, September). Emotional eating: Feeding your feelings. Retrieved from www.webmd.com.

Harding, Anne (2011, July 27). Study offers clues to emotional eating. Health. Retrieved from www.cnn.com.

Mayo Foundation for Medical Education and Research (2010, Dec. 7). Bone health, Tips to keep your bones healthy. Retrieved from www.mayoclinic.com.

Parker-Pope, Tara (2012, January 17). Obesity rates stall, but no decline. New York Times 'Well' blog. Retrieved from www.nytimes.com.

Garden-Robinson, Julie (2011, May). What color is your food? Taste a rainbow of fruits and vegetables for better health. North Dakota State University Extension Service. Retrieved from www.ag.ndsu.edu.

Zelman, Kathleen M. (2010). Weight loss and diet plans: The truth about white foods. Retrieved from www.webmd.com.

Donaldson, Michael (2012, Feb. 17). The decline in American health and a call to action. Health News Magazine. Retrieved from www.hahealthnews.com.

Haupt, Angela (2012, August 21). Study: Obesity may hasten cognitive decline. Health Buzz: U.S. News and World Report. Retrieved from www.usnews.com.

Haupt, Angela (2012, April 26). Strawberries and blueberries may stave off cognitive decline. Health Buzz: U.S. News and World Report. Retrieved from www.usnews.com

Staff report (2009, May 28). 'healthy lifestyles' wane in U.S. BBC News Online. Retrieved from http://forum.lowcarber.org.

Centers for Disease Control (2011, October 4). Nutrition for everyone: Basics. Retrieved from www.cdc.gov.

Marano, Hara (2003, Nov. 21). Stress and eating. Psychology Today. Retrieved from www.psychologytoday.com.

Kirkey, Sharon (2011, December 29). Fast food may damage your brain. Vancouver Sun. Retrieved from www.vancouversun.com.

Harvard School of Public Health Nutrition Source. Fiber: Start roughing it! Retrieved from www.hsph.harvard.edu.

Wells, Hodan; Buzby, Jean (2008, March). Dietary assessment of major trends in U.S. food consumption, 1970-2005. Economic Research Service., U.S. Department of Agriculture. Retrieved from www.ers.usda.gov.

Robinson, Joe (2011, September 14). Why comfort is actually bad for you. The Blog. Retrieved from www.huffingtonpost.com.

Ornish, Dean (2012, September 22). Eating for health, not weight. The New York Times. Retrieved from www.nytimes.com.

Joseph, James A. (2007, August). Nutrition and brain function: Food for the aging mind. Agricultural Research Service: U.S. Department of Agriculture. Retrieved from www.ars.usda.gov.

Bhanoo, Sindya (2011, January 28). How meditation may change the brain. Well blog at New York Times. Retrieved from www.nytimes.com.

Gunderson, Dan (2006, July 28). Researchers suggest link between pesticides and brain disease. Minnesota Public Radio. Retrieved from http;//minnesota.publicradio.org.

Staff report (2009, January 28). Concussion's effects may linger for decades. Health Day at U.S. News and World Report. Retrieved from www.usnews.com.

Staff report (2004, October). Alcohol alert. National Institute on Alcohol Abuse and Alcoholism. U.S. Department of Health and Human Services. Retrieved from http://pubs.niaaa.nih.gov.

Gowin, Joshua (2010, October 15). Why your brain needs water. Psychology Today. Retrieved from www.psychologytoday.com.

CHAPTER 6

Centers for Disease Control and Prevention (2012, January 17). Genomics. Retrieved from www.cdc.gov.

Deans, Emily (2011, June 26). How does diet affect symptoms of ADHD? Psychology Today. Retrieved from www.psychologytoday.com.

Genetic Science Learning Center of the University of Utah (2013). Epigenetics and the human brain. Retrieved from http://learn.genetics.utah.edu.

National Human Genome Research Institute (2011, October 19). A brief guide to genomics. Retrieved from www.genome.gov.

NOVA (2007, July 24). Epigenetics. Public Broadcasting Corporation. Retrieved from www.pbs.org.

Miller, Peter (2012, January). A thing or two about twins. National Geographic Magazine. Retrieved from http://ngm.nationalgeographic.com.

Shulevitz, Judith (2012, September 8). Why fathers really matter. The New York Times. Retrieved from www.nytimes.com.

Walton, Alice (2011, November). How healthy lifestyle choices can change your genetic make-up. The Atlantic. Retrieved from www.theatlantic.com.

Genomic Research Center (no date). Genes and human disease. World Health Organization. Retrieved form www.who.int.

University of Wisconsin Health (2011, October). Lifestyle choices can change your genes. Retrieved from www.uwhealth.org.

Sears, Al (2007, February 3). Your genetic code is not carved in stone. Retrieved from www.beinghealthynaturally.com.

Huber, Gary (2010, August 6). Want to change your genes? Just change your mind. Healthy Alter Ego. Retrieved from www.healthyalterego.com.

Lipman, Frank (2011, May 3). FAQs on epigenetics. Retrieved from www.drfranklipman.com.

CHAPTER 7

Goodman, Brenda (2011, Aug. 24). Antibiotic overuse may be bad for body's good bacteria. Retrieved from www.webmd.com.

Tanner, Lindsey (2013, Jan. 12). Flu epidemic: Hospitals crack down on workers who refuse shots. Huffpost Healthy Living. Retrieved from www.huffingtonpost.com.

Jaslow, Ryan (2013, Feb. 21). CDC: Flu vaccine only provided 9 percent protection for seniors against worst strain. CBS News. Retrieved from www.cbsnews.com.

Pediatrics & Child Health (2005, September). Facts about chickenpox. Retrieved from www.ncbi.nlm.nih.gov.

Shute, Nancy (2011, Aug. 25). Report: Vaccines are safe, hazards few and far between. National Public Radio. Retrieved from www.npr.org.

Mazo, Ellen (2011, December). The top 10 immune busters. Prevention. Retrieved from www.prevention.com.

Reader's Digest Association (2012). Four most harmful ingredients in packaged foods. Retrieved from www.rd.com.

White, Linda B. (2010, August/September). 12 strategies to strengthen your immune system. Mother Earth News. Retrieved from www.motherearthnews.com.

NutritionMD (2013). Strengthening immune function: Choose immune-boosting foods. Retrieved from www.nutritionmd.org.

Dallas, Mary Elizabeth (2013, Jan. 18). Immune-boosting foods may add to flu defense. MedlinePlus. Retrieved from www.nlm.nih.gov.

Web MD (undated). 15 immune-boosting foods. Retrieved from www.webmd.com.

Baker, Brue (undated). At last! The truth about processed food. NY Wellness Guide. Retrieved from www.nywellnessguide.com.

MacMillan, Amanda; Schryver, Tamara (2011, November). Nine power foods that boost immunity. Prevention. Retrieved from www.prevention.com.

Frontline (undated). Is your meat safe? PBS. Retrieved from www.pbs.org.

Tavernise, Sabrina (2012, Sept. 3). Farm use of antibiotics defies scrutiny. The New York Times. Retrieved from www.nytimes.com.

Hoffman, Matthew (2009). Safer food for a healthier you. WebMD. Retrieved from www.webmd.com.

Journal of Antimicrobial Chemotherapy (2004). Does the use of antibiotics in food animals pose a risk to human health? Retrieved from http://jac.oxfordjournals.org.

Dunn, Rob (2011, July 5). Scientists discover that antimicrobial wipes and soap may be making you (and society) sick. Scientific American. Retrieved from http://blogs.scientificamerican.com.

Gaines, Tyrese (undated). Will early exposure to colds boost immunity. NBC News. Retrieved from www.nbcnews.com.

McKenzie, John (2012, July 17). Antibacterial cleansers can hurt immune system. ABC News. Retrieved from http://abcnews.go.com.

CNCA Health (undated). Cold and flu: Need to know facts and myths. Retrieved from www.cncahealth.com.

Thompson, Dennis (2011). Too many meds may be more problem than cure. Health Day. Retrieved from www.usatoday.com.

Kotz: Deborah (2010, Oct. 7). Overmedication: Are Americans taking too many drugs? U.S. News & World Report. Retrieved from www.usnews.com.

Chandler, Ray (2008, Nov. 13). Don't go to the doctor during those miserable first seven days: Colds are better left untreated. Independent Mail. Retrieved from www.independentmail.com.

Kim, Ben (undated). What most doctors won't tell you about colds and flus. Dr. Ben Kim. Retrieved from http://drbenkim.com.

Moskowitz, Richard (1983, March). The case against immunizations. Journal of the AIH. Retrieved from www.homeopathyusa.org.

Live Strong (undated). What are the primary lymphoid organs? Retrieved from www.

livestrong.com.

Science Daily (undated). White blood cells. Retrieved from www.sciencedaily.com.

National Institute of Allergy and Infectious Disease (2011, April 18). Immune System. Retrieved from www.niaid.nih.gov.

University of Hartford (2001, March). Immune System. Retrieved from http://uhaweb. hartford.edu/bugl/immune.htm.

S., Jennifer (2012, Feb. 3). The anthroposophical view of feeding infants and young children. Natural Parents Network. Retrieved from http://naturalparentsnetwork.com.

Natural News (2006, Aug. 30). Anthroposophic lifestyle reduces risk of youth allergies. Retrieved from www.naturalnews.com.

Jackson, Kelly; Nazor, Andrea (2006, April). Breastfeeding, the immune response, and long-term health. Retrieved from www.ncbi.nlm.nih.gov.

Mercola, Joseph (2004, May 19). Seven reasons to breastfeed your child that you need to know. Retrieved from http://articles.mercola.com.

Brigham Young University (2008, Oct. 27). How breastfeeding transfers immunity to babies. Science Daily. Retrieved from www.sciencedaily.com.

Mayo Clinic (2012, April 10). Breast-feeding vs. formula feeding: What's best? Retrieved from www.mayoclinic.com.

Mavridara, Lilian (2009, Nov. 23). What is the difference between natural immunity and vaccine-induced immunity? Seattle Natural Health Examiner. Retrieved from www. examiner.com.

Fox, Maggie (2013, March 17). Crowded vaccine schedule for babies safe, study finds. NBC News. Retrieved from www.nbcnews.com.

Hanlon, Michael (undated). The case for and against the MMR vaccine. Daily Mail. Retrieved from www.dailymail.co.uk.

SmartVax (undated). More details on vaccine-induced asthma. Retrieved from www. smartvax.com.

National Network for Immunization Information (2004, July 19). Asthma and vaccines. Retrieved from www.immunizationinfo.org.

Brooks, Megan (2010, April 2). Early-life infections, immunizations alter childhood asthma risk. Reuters. Retrieved from www.medscape.com.

Halvorsen, Richard (2007, Nov. 9). Chickenpox vaccine is bad for children. Retrieved from www.telegraph.co.uk.

Harris, Gardiner (2011, Aug. 25). Vaccine cleared again as autism culprit. The New York Times. Retrieved from www.nytimes.com.

Park, Alice (2008, June 2). How safe are vaccines? Time. Retrieved from www.time.com.

CHAPTER 8

Dumb Little Man (undated). 14 simple ways to supercharge your brain. Retrieved from www.dumblittleman.com.

Brain Foundation (undated). The healthy brain program. Retrieved from www.brainfoundation.org.

Green, Holly (2012, March 27). How to develop five critical thinking types. Forbes. Retrieved from www.forbes.com.

Bardin, Jon (2012, Nov. 15). This is your brain on freestyle rap. Los Angeles Times. Retrieved from www.latimes.com.

Madgwick, Paul (2010, July 26). What kind of thinker are you? Retrieved from www.careernav.com.

Brown, Eryn (2011, Nov. 15). Frequent gamers have brain differences, study finds. Los Angeles Times. Retrieved form www.latimes.com.

Collins, Nick (2011, Oct. 14). Video games 'can alter children's brains.' Retrieved from www.telegraph.co.uk.

Collins, Nick (2011, Nov. 16). Children who love video games have brains like gamblers. Retrieved from www.telegrph.co.uk.

Cherry, Kendra (2012). Left brain vs. right brain. Retrieved from http://psychology.about.com.

National Institute of Health (2012, January). Breaking bad habits: Why it's so hard to change. Retrieved from http://newsinhealth.nih.gov.

Szalavitz, Maia (2012, March 2). Q & A: Charles DuHigg on changing your habits. The New York Times Magazine. Retrieved from http://healthland.time.com.

Hamilton, Jon (2010, April 15). Brain maxes out at multitasking. National Public Radio. Retrieved from www.npr.org.

Sundem, Garth (2012, Feb. 24). This is your brain on multitasking. Psychology Today. Retrieved from www.psychologytoday.com.

Science Daily (2010, Sept. 10). Biofeedback for your brain? Retrieved from www.sciencedaily.com.

Curley, Ann J. (2012, Jan. 18). Study: Challenging seniors' brains can also change their personality. CNN. Retrieved from www.cnn.com.

Boyd, Robynne (2008, Feb. 7). Do people only use 10 percent of their brains? Scientific American. Retrieved from www.scientificamerican.com.

Zelinski, Elizabeth (2010, April 8). Brain maintenance: Cognitive enhancement first, Alzheimer's delay second. Retrieved from www.sharpbrains.com.

Science Daily (2012, April 27). Maintain your brain: The secrets to aging success. Retrieved from www.sciencedaily.com.

Ault, Alicia (2006, Feb. 21). Preventive maintenance for the brain. The Washington Post. Retrieved from www.washingtonpost.com.

Ingall, Richard (2010). Why changes of routine can help prevent depression. Jekyll & Hyde Publishing. Retrieved from www.depressionbeater.com.

Sargent, Betty Kelly (2010, Feb. 2). Change your brain, change your routine, change your life. Retrieved from www.tipsonhealthyliving.com.

Science Daily (2006, May 22). Simple lifestyle changes may improve cognitive function and brain efficiency. Retrieved from www.sciencedaily.com.

Posit Science (2012). Brain mythology. Retrieved from www.positscience.com.

American Health Assistance Foundation (2012, Oct. 4). Anatomy of the brain. Retrieved from www.ahaf.org.

American Association of Neurological Surgeons (2006, June). Anatomy of the brain. Retrieved from www.aans.org.

Levinson, Daniel (2012, March 15). A wandering mind reveals mental processes and priorities. University of Wisconsin-Madison. Retrieved from www.eurekaalert.org.

Duke Health (2011, Jan. 18). Brain's 'autopilot' provides insight into early development of Alzheimer's disease. Neurology. Retrieved from www.dukehealth.org.

Rock, David (2010, Nov. 14). New study shows humans are on autopilot nearly half the time. Psychology Today. Retrieved from www.psychologytoday.com.

NBC News (2010, Feb. 10). Can you really be bored to death? Retrieved from www.nbcnews.com.

Kashdan, Todd (201, March 3). Science shows you can die of boredom, literally. Psychology Today. Retrieved from www.psychologytoday.com.

Reynolds, Susan (2011, July 14). Is your brain asleep on the job. Psychology Today. Retrieved form www.psychologytoday.com.

Spiegel, Alix (2009, March 12). Bored? Try doodling to keep the brain on task. National Public Radio. Retrieved from www.npr.org.

Gazzaley, Adam (2012, Sept. 23). How mobile tech can influence our brain. CNN. Retrieved from www.cnn.com.

CHAPTER 9

Collins, Nick (2012, Jan. 11). Alcohol releases addictive endorphins, study shows. Retrieved from www.telegraph.co.uk.

Soppler, Melissa Conrad (2007, March 15). Endorphins: Natural pain and stress fighters. Retrieved from www.medicinenet.com.

Conger, Krista (2003, Dec. 10). Laughter, like drugs, tickles brain's reward center. Stanford Report. Retrieved from http://news.stanford.edu.

Welsh, Jennifer (2011, Sept. 14). Why laughter may be the best pain medicine. Scientific American. Retrieved from www.scientificamerican.com.

Holt, Doug (2008, Jan. 8). The role of the amygdala in fear and panic. Serendip Studio. Retrieved http://serendip.brynmawr.edu.

Beard, Emily (undated). What do emotions have to do with brain development? Retrieved from www.creatingconnectionsic.com.

Black, Harvey (2001, Oct. 1). Amygdala's inner workings. The Scientist. Retrieved from www.biopsychiatroy.com.

Szalavitz, Maia (2010, Dec. 28). How to win friends: Have a big amygdala? Time. Retrieved from http://healthland.time.com.

Swenson, Rand (2006). Review of clinical and functional neuroscience. Dartmouth University. Retrieved from www.dartmouth.edu.

Harris, Dan; Brady, Erin (2011, July 28). Rewiring your brain for happiness: Research shows how meditation can physically change the brain. ABC News. Retrieved from http://abcnews.go.com.

Hanson, Rick (2011, Sept. 26). How to trick your brain for happiness. Retrieved from www.greatergood.berkeley.edu.

Yount, Kathleen (2007). The geography of happiness. University of Alabama at Birmingham. Retrieved from http://main.uab.edu.

Smith, Melida; Kemp, Gina; Segal, Jeanne (2012, November). Laughter is the best medicine. Helpguide. Retrieved from www.helpguide.org.

Gustafson, Timi (2012, Nov. 14). The many health benefits of a good belly laugh. Huffington Post. Retrieved from www.huffingtonposts.com.

Marano, Hara Estroff (undated). The benefits of laughter. Psychology Today. Retrieved form www.psychologytoday.com.

Kringelback, Morten L. (2006, May 2). Searching the brain for happiness. BBC News. Retrieved from http://newsvote.bbc.co.uk.

Reynolds, Susan (2011, Aug. 2). Happy brain, happy life. Psychology Today. Retrieved from www.psychologytoday.com.

Goleman, Daniel (1995, March 28). The brain manages happiness and sadness in different centers. The New York Times. Retrieved from www.nytimes.com.

Bolton, Jane (2010, May 20). Crying for mental health? Psychology Today. Retrieved from www.psychologytoday.com.

Thompson, Dennis Jr. (undated). Is crying healthy? Everyday Health. Retrieved from www.everydayhealth.com.

Gorman, Rachael Moeller (2010, May/June). New science links food and happiness. Eating Well. Retrieved from www.eatingwell.com.

Trei, Lisa (2002, July 10). Happy faces trigger different brain reactions in extroverts and introverts. Stanford University. Retrieved from http://news.stanford.edu.

Stillman, Jessica (2012, Feb. 27). Happiness makes your brain work better. Inc. magazine. Retrieved from www.inc.com.

Lyon, Lindsay (2009, June 24). Positive psychology. U.S. News & World Report. Retrieved from http://health.usnews.com.

Dahl, Melissa (2008, Dec. 4). Your happiness could be contagious. MSNBC. Retrieved from www.msnbc.com.

Goode, Erica (2003, Sept. 2). Power of positive thinking may have a health benefit, study says. The New York Times. Retrieved from www.nytimes.com.

Neergaard, Lauran (2012, April 17). Happy? Positive outlook may be good for your heart. USA Today. Retrieved from http://usatoday30.usatoday.com.

Cherry, Kendra (undated). Benefits of positive thinking. Retrieved from http://psychology.about.com.

Waldman, Mark; Newberg, Andrew (2012, July 31). The most dangerous word in the world. Psychology Today. Retrieved form www.psychologytoday.com.

Live Science (2008, March). Happiness is partly inherited. Retrieved from www.livescience.com.

Herper, Matthew (2004, Sept. 23). Happiness is mostly genetic. Forbes. Retrieved from www.forbes.com.

Sigman, Michael (2011, Sept. 28). The genetic reason some of us are happier. Huffington Post. Retrieved from www.huffingtonpost.com

Merkin, Daphne (2012, July 28). Is depression inherited? The New York Times. Retrieved from www.nytimes.com.

Coyle, Daniel (2012, Dec. 11). The most powerful three-letter word a parent can use. Retrieved from http://thetalentcode.com.

Coyle, Daniel (2009). The Talent Code. Bantam.

Marano, Hara Estroff (2003, June 20). Our brain's negative bias. Psychology Today. Retrieved from www.psychologytoday.com.

CHAPTER 10

Science Daily (2009, Nov. 30). Therapeutic benefits of the human-animal bond. Retrieved from www.sciencedaily.com.

Rovner, Julie (2012, Marc 5). Pet therapy: How animals and humans heal each other. National Public Radio. Retrieved from www.npr.org.

National Institute of Health (2009, February). Can pets help keep you healthy? NIH News in Health. Retrieved from www.newsinhealth.nih.gov.

National Center for Infectious Disease (2010, July 28). Healthy pets healthy people. CDC. Retrieved from www.cdc.gov.

Discovery Health (undated). Furry friends can aid your health. Retrieved from http://health.howstuffworks.com.

McConnell, Allen R. (2011, July 11). Friends with benefits: Pets make us happier, healthier. Psychology Today. Retrieved from www.psychologytoday.com.

Nauert, Rick (2012, Aug. 3). Close relationships influence health, happiness. PsychCentral. Retrieved from http://psychcentral.com.

North, Kat (2012, Sept. 11). How does divorce affect children? Cary, N.C. Citizen. Retrieved from www.carycitizen.com.

Valeo, Tom (2007, January). Good friends are good for you. WebMd. Retrieved from www.webmd.com.

Center for Disease Control and Prevent (2010, Jan. 25). Family environment affects health of family members. Retrieved from www.cdc.gov.

Mayo Clinic (2011, April 16). Friendships: Enrich your life and improve your health. Retrieved from www.mayoclinic.com.

Gill, Victoria (2012, Dec. 28). Kinder children are more popular. BBC News. Retrieved from www.bbc.co.uk.

Sample, Ian (2010, July 27). With a little help from your friends you can live longer. The Guardian. Retrieved from www.guardian.co.uk.

Casserly, Meghan (2010, Aug. 24). Friends with health benefits. Forbes. Retrieved from www.forbes.com.

Parker-Pope, Tara (2009, April 21). What are friends for? A longer life. The New York Times. Retrieved from www.nytimes.com.

Dembling, Sophia (2010, May 13). You've got to have friends, but how many? Psychology Today. Retrieved from www.psychologytoday.com.

Cohen, Sheldon (2004, November). Social relationships and health. American Psychologist. Retrieved from www.apa.org.

Doyle, Terrence A. (2005, Jan. 19). Types of interpersonal relationships. Retrieved from http://novaonline.nvcc.edu.

Harvard Health Publications (2010, December). The health benefits of strong relationships. Retrieved from http://health.harvard.edu.

Kansas State University Counseling Services (2000). Healthy relationships. Retrieved from www.k-state.edu.

Marano, Hara Estroff (undated). What is solitude? Psychology Today. Retrieved from www.psychologytoday.com.

Cherry, Kendra (undated). Loneliness. Retrieved from http://psychology.about.com.

Marche, Stephen (2013). Is Facebook making us lonely? The Atlantic. Retrieved from www.theatlantic.com.

Cacioppo, John T. (2009, May 3). Epidemic of loneliness. Psychology Today. Retrieved from www.psychologytoday.com.

Warrell, Maria (2012, Oct. 23). Is technology making you lonely? Forbes. Retrieved from www.forbes.com.

Jaksch, Mary (undated). How to escape loneliness. Goodlife Zen. Retrieved from http://goodlifezen.com.

Kozlowski, Lori (2012, April 25). The seven pillars of connecting with absolutely anyone. Forbes. Retrieved from www.forbes.com.

Lyubomirsky, Sonja (undated). Connect with others. Retrieved from www.liveyourlifewell.org.

PsyBlog (2007, July). Empathy causes facial similarities between couples to increase over time. Retrieved from www.spring.org.uk.

PsyBlog (2007, April). Seven signs of relationship (dis)satisfaction. Retrieved from www.spring.org.uk.

McAllister, Rallie (2007). Arguing with your spouse could be hazardous to your health. Creators Syndicate. Retrieved from www.creators.com.

Roan, Shar (2011, May 5). Spouses affect each other's health dramatically, study finds. Los Angeles Times. Retrieved from www.latimes.com.

Sutton, Robert (2010, July 25). The fine art of emotional detachment. Psychology Today. Retrieved from www.psychologytoday.com.

Lynch, Carmen (2000). Patterns of relationships. Retrieved from www.sonoma.edu.

CHAPTER 11

Larson, Christine (2008, Dec. 22). Health prayer: Should religion and faith have roles in medicine? U.S. News & World Report. Retrieved from www.usnews.com.

Larson, Christine (2008, Dec. 22). Say two Hail Marys, and call me in the morning. U.S. News & World Report. Retrieved from www.usnews.com.

University of Maryland Medical Center (undated). Spirituality. Retrieved from www.umm.edu.

Friedman, Howard S. (undated). How prayer leads to better health and longer life. Huffington Post. Retrieved from www.huffingtonpost.com.

Mayo Clinic (2010, July 23). Spirituality and stress relief: Make the connection. Retrieved from www.mayoclinic.com.

Dartmouth-Hitchcock Medical Center (2011, Sept. 12). Can religious, spiritual beliefs affect health? Retrieved from www.dartmouth-hitchcock.org.

Stosny, Steven (2012, Oct. 12). Resentment in marriage. Psychology Today. Retrieved from www.psychologytoday.com.

Feldscher, Karen (2011, Aug. 15). Take it to heart: Positive emotions may be good for health. Harvard School of Public Health. Retrieved from www.hsph.harvard.edu.

Wilson, Tobi; Milosevic, Aleks; Carroll, Michelle; Hart, Kenneth; Hibbard, Stephen (2008, Aug. 12). Physical health status in relation to self-forgiveness and other-forgiveness in healthy college students. Journal of Health Psychology. Retrieved from www.hpq.sagepub.com.

Gottesman, Nancy (2011, April). Are happy people healthier? Oprah Magazine. Retrieved from www.oprah.com.

Stosny, Steven (2011, Aug. 5). Overcoming chronic resentment and the abuse it causes. Psychology Today. Retrieved from www.psychologytoday.com.

Huffington Post Religion (2010, June 16). The science of forgiveness. The Huffington Post. Retrieved from www.huffingtonpost.com.

Dotinga, Randy (2008, Feb. 8). Mutual resentment in marriage can be deadly. Health Day News. Retrieved from http://news.healingwell.com.

Healy, Melissa (2007, Dec. 31). Forgive and be well? Los Angeles Times. Retrieved from www.latimes.com.

Institute for Social Research (2001, Dec. 11). How link between forgiveness and health changes with age. Retrieved from www.ns.umich.edu.

Brown, Harriet (2011, April 27). How to forgive others. OWN TV. Retrieved from www.oprah.com.

Mayo Clinic (2011, Nov. 23). Forgiveness: Letting go of grudges and bitterness. Retrieved from www.mayoclinic.com.

Banschick, Mark (2011, Oct. 3). Can you forgive? Psychology Today. Retrieved from www.psychologytoday.com.

Haupt, Angela (2012, Aug. 29). How to forgive, and why you should. U.S. News & World Report. Retrieved from www.usnews.com.

Klimes, R (undated). Forgiveness methods. Retrieved from www.psychologytools.org.

Worthington, Everett L. (2004, fall). The new science of forgiveness. The Greater Good Science Center. Retrieved from http://greatergood.berkeley.edu.

Stonsy, Steven (2009, April 9). Marriage problems: Resentment and the decline of interest. Psychology Today. Retrieved from www.psychologytoday.com.

MacMillan, Amanda (2011, Oct. 4). Depressed brains may hate differently. CNN. Retrieved from www.cnn.com.

Paetzold, Ramona (2012, July 5). Mindfulness links forgiveness to better health. Retrieved from www.examiner.com.

Heartland Forgiveness Scale (2013). Retrieved from www.heartlandforgiveness.com.

Gordon, Bennet (2009, June 11). Forgiveness is healthy. Huffington Post. Retrieved from www.huffingtonpost.com.

Hough, Andrew (2010, Oct. 6). Having faith 'helps patients live longer,' study suggests. Retrieved from www.telegraph.co.uk.

The Creative Trust (undated). Seven characteristics of a spiritual person. Retrieved from www.creativetrust.com.

Dyer, Jade (2007). How does spirituality affect physical health? Holistic Nurse Practitioner.

Moore, Thomas (2011, March-April). Being a spiritual person. Spirituality & Health Magazine. Retrieved from http://spiritualityhealth.com.

CHAPTER 12

Mayo Foundation for Medical Research and Education (2008). Weight maintenance: Keep the weight off permanently. Retrieved from www.cnn.com.

Ipaktchian, Susan (2012, Oct. 30). Mastering weight-maintenance skills before embarking on diet helps women avoid backsliding, study shows. Stanford School of Medicine. Retrieved from http://med.stanford.edu.

Holland, Veronica (2012, Nov. 26). Experts advise holiday weight maintenance, not weight loss. ABC News. Retrieved from http://abcnews.go.com.

Roan, Shari (2010, Nov. 24). Study identifies foods that promote weight maintenance. Los Angeles Times. Retrieved from www.latimes.com.

Halvorson, Heidi Grant (2011, April 4). The science of success. Psychology Today. Retrieved from www.psychologytoday.com

Knaus, Bill (2012, Nov. 19). Harness your imagination to break bad habits. Psychology

Today. Retrieved from www.psychologytoday.com.

National Institute of Health (2012, January). Breaking bad habits: Why it's so hard to change. NIH News in Health. Retrieved from http://newsinhealth.nih.gov.

Dallas South News (2013, March 19). Three ways to push past workout plateaus. Retrieved from www.dallassouthnews.org.

Harvard Medical School (undated). Special Health Report: Exercise – A program you can live with. Retrieved from www.health.harvard.edu.

Shaw, Gina (2009, July 10). Have you hit a fitness plateau? WebMD. Retrieved from www.webmd.com.

Dale, Heather (2011, Nov. 10). How to know if you've hit a fitness plateau and what to do about it. FitSugar. Retrieved from http://news.health.com.

Fit Day (undated). Why you should change up your workout routine daily. Retrieved from www.fitday.com.

Mathews, Joy Pierce (2011, Jan. 10). Tips for maintaining a successful exercise routine. Summit Medical Group. Retrieved from www.summitmedicalgroup.com.

Thompson, Jonathan (2012, April 12). Avoiding training pleateaus. Livestrong. Retrieved from www.livestrongfitness.com.

Sears, Barry (undated). Maintaining a healthy brain. The Christian Broadcasting Network. Retrieved from www.cbn.com.

Reader's Digest (2012). Seven anti-aging tips to keep your brain young. Retrieved from www.rd.com.

Center for Disease Control and Prevention (2011, Aug. 31). Healthy brain initiative. Retrieved from www.cdc.gov.

Open Education Database (2013, Feb. 26). Brain power: 100 ways to keep your mind healthy and fit. Retrieved from http://oedb.org.

INDEX

D

E

N

O

P

Q

R

S